What others are saying about *Annibalism: Vegan Solutionaries Rising*

"*Annibalism* filled me with a sense of calm and purpose. Reading Dean's book reminded me of the core reasons I became, and have stayed, vegan. His book has given me tools and strength to continue teaching others all of the reasons why we need to aim for a kinder, vegan world. Compassion is key. To everything we do."

Lea McBride – Vegan Festival Adelaide Director

* *

"Dean gets straight to the heart of the vegan lifestyle with *Anniblaism*, making it simple and accessible. He has navigated the difficult task of honestly addressing the horror of what is currently happening to the animals we share this world with, without ever veering into bleakness or despair – instead leaving us with as profoundly hope-filled and peaceful outlook, and solid steps we can take to be of aid. I hope this book finds its way into the hands of everyone who needs it. I really appreciate the wisdom and research that has gone into this book, and how much love shines through every page."

This book is such a 'work of heart'

Kimberley Deeney – vegan parent and earth mother

* * *

"Finally, the book the world needs about veganism as a spiritual practice! This book resonated with me deeply because it unapologetically embraces compassion as the number one reason to go vegan. The author, Dean Rees-Evans, discusses several important reasons, but ultimately the premise is that animals are sentient and they don't want to die.

The book is filled with thoughtful anecdotes about Dean's experiences with animals, which reveal their emotional intelligence, wisdom and how animals are just like us in all the ways that matter. This book is an insightful read because it's easy to sometimes get angry about what happens to animals – angry at industries, businesses and consumers.

But in *Anniblaism* it is lovingly pointed out that consistent compassion is the only way forward. The same compassion we give freely to animals, we have to share with humans, too, because so much of our behaviour as humans is conditioned and innocent. I loved that this point was strongly made. It's only with a clear mind and good mental health that we can help animals in a lasting way. Amen! This work is a gift to animals and humans alike."

Avleen Masawan – Copywriter and Sydney based Author

* * *

"In this book Dean Rees-Evans gives a thoughtful and refreshing take on veganism as a celebration of life, a spiritual act of compassion, and respect for both oneself and all living beings. More importantly, he explores the physical and mental wellbeing of those seeking to undertake this noble and self-transformative, but easily undertaken, practice. It is my belief that the world, perhaps more than ever, is in deep need of the love and compassion of which veganism is an expression."

Dhammakumara - Chairman of Sydney Buddhist Centre

*   *   *

"Becoming vegan means going on a journey, physically, mentally, emotionally and spiritually. Like any journey of exploration, it helps to have a guidebook written by an experienced traveller who can point out both the important landmarks and the hidden pitfalls. Dean Rees-Evans' book is just such a guidebook. Keep it close by as you begin your vegan journey and dip back into it as you move through the stages. In particular, heed Dean's wise words on reconnecting with your innate mental health by tuning into the wisdom of your own quiet mind. This simple yet profound practice will not only help you be a happier vegan, but a far more effective change agent in a world that needs this, more than anything."

Robyn Chuter BHSc(Hons), ND, GDCouns, FASLM, MATMS
ASLM Certified Lifestyle Medicine Practitioner

*   *   *

"Dean has written a book not unlike himself, quietly spoken, clear, healthy, and compassionate; a great exploration of veganism – its roots, impacts and angles – from the very personal to the very real global perspectives. A great read for understanding yourself, your relationship to food and animals, our planet and all the beings that share it. The large scale changes we are seeing are worth everyone's understanding and attention because it's evolution, Baby!"

Jennie Fenton – Councillor, Bellingen Shire Council

* * *

"*Annibalism* is exceptionaly informative and insightfully brilliant as it expresses fresh perspectives on a variety of topics. It leaves one engaged, encouraged and inspired to rise to the compassionate solutions that Dean speaks of. I loved this book in all its entirety."

Tracey Chapman
Animal rights Advocate,
Spiritual and Wellbeing Practitioner

* * *

"*Annibalism* provides the facts about what is happening to animals in the world, but also encourages the reader to be positive about the changes the individual can make by becoming vegan. For me, after eight years being vegan, this book has realigned my values and given me hope that we are at the beginning of a huge shift in peoples awareness and an increase in compassion for all living beings."

Anne Bates
Solutionary
BBus, CPA

* * *

"*Annibalism* is full of insight, easy to read and relatable to both vegans and non-vegans alike. I was drawn into the wisdom that has echoed throughout the decades. A wonderful book for any bookshelf and would certainly make a great gift for any non vegan seeking a more loving and peaceful existence, without violence to our beautiful animal cousins."

Flavia Ursino Coleman
Poet, and author of *Beyond Speciesism*, and co-author of *Monkey Business: A Story of Soulmates and Primates*

* * *

"This book is a treasure trove of applied ancient wisdom and personal leadership whilst offering a practical roadmap to create a compassionate, abundant and creative world. Its grasp is within our hands - through a personal journey of ethical veganism, re-discovering the solution to our problems we have somehow chosen to forget".

Clare Mann
Author of *Vystopia: The Anguish of Being Vegan in a Non Vegan World*

* * *

annibalism

Vegan Solutionaries Rising

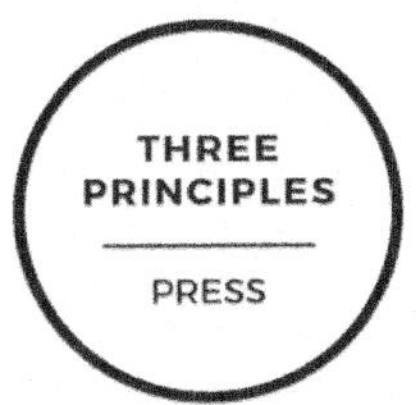

Published by Three Principles Press

All enquires to ThreePrinciplesPress@gmail.com

Cover Design: Izii_Designer

Editing: Naomi Elliot and Tom Rothsey

ISBN 978-0-6457164-0-5 (Paperback)

ISBN 978-0-6457164-1-2 (e-book)

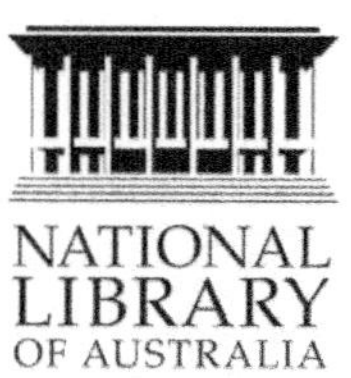

A catalogue record of this work is available from the National Library of Australia

Table of Contents

Dedication

I dedicate this book to all the brave souls that give their voice to the voiceless and their daily endeavours to alleviate the suffering of innocent beauty of this world; and to all those who work tirelessly against the tyranny of speciesism in all its abhorrent forms. Heroes to the last.

Love, life and liberty for all living creatures is our endgame.

Creon: "An enemy is still an enemy. Dead or alive."

Antigone: "No, I was born with love enough to share: no hate for anyone."

From Antigone by Sophocles

"This is what you shall do; Love the earth and sun and the animals, despise riches, give alms to every one that asks, stand up for the stupid and crazy, devote your income and labor to others, hate tyrants, argue not concerning God, have patience and indulgence toward the people, take off your hat to nothing known or unknown or to any man or number of men, go freely with powerful uneducated persons and with the young and with the mothers of families, read these leaves in the open air every season of every year of your life, re-examine all you have been told at school or church or in any book, dismiss whatever insults your own soul, and your very flesh shall be a great poem and have the richest fluency not only in its words but in the silent lines of its lips and face and between the lashes of your eyes and in every motion and joint of your body".

Walt Whitman (1819–1892)

Foreword

What sort of world will our children inherit from us?

With every passing day, it seems to become more obvious: the mentality that underlies our culture's socio-economic system is destroying the biodiversity and ecological integrity of our earth, poisoning human health and damaging communities and relationships. This underlying mentality is mandated and continually reinforced by our culture's daily meals, in which we're taught as children to disconnect from animals and the suffering we cause them, and to see them as mere commodities. We are taught to eat like predators, and the industrialized factory farms and slaughter plants permeating our culture are actually systematized predatory mechanisms that have co-evolved with other predatory mechanisms—the massive corporations and financial institutions that prey on the earth, animals, and vulnerable people being one example. Our meals and institutions reflect each other and reinforce the delusion that we are violent and competitive by nature.

Spiritual and religious teachings say otherwise. The Bodhisattva ideal that Buddhists emulate, as but one example, embodies the understanding that our true nature is wisdom, loving-kindness and cooperativeness. Our greatest joy comes in helping others and blessing them, and we hurt ourselves the most when we harm others for our own gain. The Golden Rule is universally recognized as essential in all the wisdom traditions of the world, and yet this universal understanding has been suppressed in our culture, and we find the predatory violence of our daily meals projected in technologically magnified ways as cluster bombs, universal wiretapping, genetic engineering, whale-killing sonar blasts, and the commodification of the Earth and her inhabitants.

It's becoming obvious that our culture's predatory mentality is blindly self-destructive. As the author Dean Rees-Evans makes clear, veganism is ancient wisdom whose time has come—with urgency! Though the word vegan is relatively new—coined in 1944 by Donald Watson—the idea behind it goes back many centuries. I lived in a Zen monastery in Korea, for example, where people had been practicing veganism for over 600 years, following a tradition going back at least 2,500 years—eating no animal-sourced foods, wearing no animal-sourced clothes, and practicing nonviolence to other beings for ethical reasons.

This ancient idea of veganism is a transformative balm to our culture's wounds, and there is nothing more essential we can do than contribute to its propagation, and nothing more healing to our world than to be practicing vegans. Veganism is the essence of inclusiveness and nonviolence: seeing sacred beings when we see others, and never reducing them to objects or commodities for our use.

Our culture's dilemmas mount because our cultural mentality is obsolete. Our technology boosts this outmoded mentality in its task of predation and thereby reinforces it. Powerful high-tech weapons, bulldozers, fishing fleets, and surveillance systems are obvious examples of this. There are countless ways we oppress and abuse animals, and if our culture doesn't evolve to the vegan ethic of compassion to all beings, and continues to use and prey on animals, our technology will magnify our violence and we'll do the same to each other.

Veganism, based on our intuitive understanding of the interconnectedness of the welfare of all, is also the dawning mentality that is foundational to sustainability, freedom, and lasting peace. May we succeed in fully digesting, contemplating, and aligning our lives with the wisdom in this compact and potent book, and share it with others. Our children's world will be vegan, or the alternative is unpleasant to contemplate.

Will Tuttle, Ph.D., visionary educator, musician, and Zen priest, is author of the international bestseller, *The World Peace Diet*, published in 16 languages, and is cofounder of Karuna Music & Art and the Worldwide Prayer Circle for Animals.

Preface

This book was first conceived as a tiny seed right at the beginning of my vegan journey. Later it grew into a small tree and began to produce fruit. It started to become more and more obvious to me that this wonderful spiritual journey that I had taken was worth sharing with others. It is my hope that people will find value and appeal in it and glean insights into the nature of living compassionately. What struck me deeply was the profoundly spiritual significance of this small act of becoming a vegan.

As my tree grew and I began to eat the fruit it offered. It became apparent to me that my idea for this book was somewhat unique in its approach to a person's decision to become a vegan. I realised that the effect of sharing my experience in this way, created the potential to initiate a profound shift in consciousness for the reader. At the very least it could have a marked impression upon the individual looking to become vegan. This experience was for me, such a significant and profound event in my life, that I felt it was worth sharing enough to warrant the book that you now read.

The turning point of full commitment to this project came while I was giving a short talk for another vegan author in Sydney. This was at the launch of one of her books, and a number of us spoke at the event on her behalf. I was so excited after giving my presentation, that I pestered the busy author, during this launch, into a conversation about my idea, and was given great support, encouragement and enthusiasm to get on with it. So, many years later, here it is.

If you are a vegan, or thinking of becoming a vegan you may well have arrived at the right book at the right time, and there really is no better time to start than now. As an ancient adage goes: *"The opportunity of a lifetime, must be taken during the lifetime of the opportunity"*. The world needs this, the animals need this, and you will be doing so much greatness by becoming vegan, which will take little effort at all. The impact of this one act is as far reaching as we can contemplate or begin to imagine. Take a running jump at this golden opportunity to turn things around in the world. You may well be the very person the world has been waiting for. With all your unique ideas and creativities that emanate from who you really are, to become the individual that changes things forever. At the very least your impact in making this decision will be far greater than you can imagine.

I encourage you to come on this journey with me; I believe it to be one of the most magical steps you will take in this brief life of ours.

Happy reading, I wish you health, happiness and a long and compassionate life of magic and wonder.

Dean Rees-Evans MSc

March 2023

Introduction

This is not a standard or comprehensive 'How to become a vegan' style of book. It is more of an analysis of what it means to be vegan. I believe that veganism is about celebrating the gift of life, because living as a vegan, stands in opposition to the taking of life. Additionally, I believe that being vegan is not simply a lifestyle choice, but moreover, it is a positive act of defiance against all animal suffering, and their cruel and needless slaughter.

With great power, it is said, comes great responsibility. However, I would like to argue that moreover, with the great vulnerability, delicacy and innocence of our animal cousins, there comes an even greater responsibility to defend, protect and love them. For, without the insistent demand of life to shield, guard, and preserve the voiceless innocent, we become less than human.

As you pick up this book and browse it, you may be wondering about the title? In many respects it came about as the direct result of my own journey into veganism. When I was a child, I was what you might call a very fussy eater. There weren't many foods that I actually liked and so this made it very difficult for my parents. Nevertheless, I survived my early years, on a 'not so healthy diet', and made it through to my early teens where I continued my abhorrence of meat. One day while looking pitifully at my dinner plate (probably a so-called traditional Sunday roast), I happened to notice that there were veins that had been dissected during the slicing of the meat. All my life I have had very healthy and prominent looking veins; nurses have often commented how easy it is to take blood samples from me. However, in this instance, looking at what lay in front of me on my plate, I felt so disgusted at the sight of these veins on my plate that I simply couldn't eat any more of the stuff. It made me think that this was like cannibalism. How could we do this, how could people not see how wrong this was, to kill and to eat our dear and beautiful cousins of the animal kingdom? How was it different from eating each other? It made no sense to me, and helped me to understand my lifelong revulsion of eating flesh.

I had to come up with a plan, and fast. Our pet dog Toby became my best friend. He ate with great enthusiasm, all the meat that slipped from my plate into his waiting and eager mouth. Success! It was a 'eureka' moment for me. I had conquered the demon of being forced to eat what was to me vile, disgusting, and unacceptable as food. Unfortunately, my stepmother noticed that our pet dog stopped eating his tinned dog food. Thus, our lovely dog was banned from the dining room (and I can only assume that he was as upset about the arrangement as I was), so I had to come up with an even more cunning plan, and I did! Each night as we were called to table for dinner, I would rush to the bathroom and proceed to fill my pocket with toilet tissue, lots of toilet tissue. Once at the dinner table, and left to: "eat up and hurry about it" as the command was made each night, I would slip all my unwanted dead animal into the tissue paper, wrap it up, and place it back into my pocket. Then, after dinner, I would ceremoniously flush it down the toilet. In my opinion this was the best place for it, if the poor dog was going to be denied, then it must be disposed of in the most efficient way, leaving no trace at all. Oh, what a joy it was to be free from being forced to become the living graveyard of all those innocent and beautiful creatures that had been killed in my name. I hasten to add; this killing was done without my consent. Thus, my early teen memories of this time in my life, turned from the term 'cannibalism' to what I felt it really was: 'annibalism'. That flesh was flesh, whether it came from a friend in the human world or from a friend in the animal world. I couldn't see how we had made this alarming distinction between the two. Thus, I coined the term, created my own dictionary definition for it, and my title was born.

I don't actually remember how long the gap was, but eventually the toilet paper being used up at a higher rate than was considered normal came into question. Thankfully, the linking between the toilet paper going down at an alarming rate, and my unwanted meat from my dinner plate being ceremoniously flushed down the toilet was never made. Phew! What a relief.

The main theme of this book is the idea that becoming vegan is a highly significant and spiritual act of deepest compassion, with the power to transform the individual making this transition. The topics covered are varied and include *how* being a vegan can realistically be understood, including my own journey to this wonderful place. It explores the doubts that sometimes arise for people in making this switch to a life of compassion. The multifaceted reasons people decide to become vegan and what that might mean. As vegans, whom do we find ourselves among in the history of compassion? The ever-growing industry that is addressing the rising need for vegan products, services, foods and beverages. The book also explores the simple fact that becoming vegan is *not* about the renunciation of a good life. Nor is it one of self-denial. It is in fact, a path that leads to the development of warmest compassion and a freeing up of all that is good in us. Veganism is a celebration of the whole of life and all the beings we share this beautiful planet with.

Additionally, the book explores the necessity of positive physical and mental health and wellbeing as the platform and foundation for a good life. And in making these endeavours towards good health, we become more capable of doing the most good for our animal cousins in the time allotted to us on earth. The book reviews the power of *Thought* and how it can be harnessed to do so much more good in the world than anger and hatred ever could. This is due to the fact that love and hate cannot coexist in the same space at the same time. The book surveys how deeply buried our society's ideas of food are; and how we can begin to see past the illusion of our culture. Long held traditions and the current status quo around animal products and meat consumption are touched on. The book also looks at the issue of human induced Environmental devastation.

Furthermore, the book reviews the simple fact that food is life, and how *no* animal life needs to be taken to sustain humanity for its health. The book takes a brief look at animal behaviour, in an attempt to more fully understand our mutual commonalities. The book looks at what some farmers and ex-farmers have to say about animals. Additionally, it also explores the many hidden layers of speciesism, and why most people seem to be blind to its presence in the modern world, and ultimately their part in it. A brief look into the historical changes that have preceded us, and the hope this can bring us, is considered. Especially when we see what difficulties these heroic figures faced in their day, and what impact their work is still having, down through the centuries to today.

The book touches briefly on the topics of drugs, tobacco and alcohol in the context of veganism. We also take a journey into the Joy we can witness of young and vibrant animal life, and how it expresses itself. Additionally, exploring the idea of looking at veganism as a natural part of evolution for our species. Also addressing the damaging consequences of slaughterhouse work on the individual, their families, and society in general. The connection between being vegan and the alleviation of starvation in developing countries is looked at. Vivisection: the dark side to protecting humans from harm is touched upon briefly. And one further topic of contention, which is explored, are pets, and what responsibilities come with the guardianship of ‘owning’ an animal.

What does it mean to become a Vegan?

"The thinking [hu]man must oppose all cruel customs no matter how deeply rooted in tradition or surrounded by a halo . . . We need a boundless ethic which will include the animals also." Dr. Albert Schweitzer (1875–1965)

The first thing I would like to share with you is this: the only way a person can truly and fully understand what it means to be a vegan is by becoming one. This may seem obvious at first glance, but because of the transformation and evolution that takes place within, this shift in consciousness can never be understood through words alone. It is a lived experience that can only be vaguely comprehended by a person that is not yet a vegan. I have read and listened to philosophical discussions about the topic of eating animals, and I have often found that those that argue for the eating of flesh, for whatever reason, really do seem to be missing the point in terms of the ethics of the issue. In my opinion, no amount of philosophising can take away the necessity that in order to eat meat, one must first take life. Therein lies the fundamental problem. The taking of life, the very gift we are given to live out and enjoy to our fullest capacity, is always going to be wrong in all contexts. All life is sacred, and therefore demands our protection, support and love.

So as you read this book, please don't take my word for it. Try it out for yourself and see where it ultimately leads. I truly and passionately believe that a purity of being arises within us on taking this simple step, which has no comparison in the world whatsoever. We can of course, given time, cover over this beautiful feeling and experience with layer upon layer of acquired thinking from others in the world. This may lead to the fading of the utter bliss and imperative importance of this one huge act of compassion, but when our mind is still, it is easy to remember why we became vegan. And how very simple it is to become and remain vegan in the modern world. There are vegan products and foods easily and readily available from almost every store you care to name. In fact all naturally grown food is vegan, bar animal products themselves. And most non-vegan establishments worth their salt usually have vegan options available. In fact, in the past few years, large corporations are tripping over themselves to get a slice of the ever growing 'vegan pie', especially in terms of producing plant-based foods, meals and beverages. Veganism is on the rise globally and as a Google search term it scores extremely high among the most popular searches out there.

The day I became vegan was one of the most noteworthy days of my life. I didn't realise it until the actual day, and then it hit me hard! This was one of the most significant things I could decide to do with my life. It was a huge ethical step and an enormous spiritual shift. I could not put it into words at the time, but I felt it deeply within the very core of my being, in every fibre of my body. It was like I woke up from a long dream of suffering. And upon waking, I knew that this decision had enormous consequences for all the lives that would no longer be taken in my name.

So, this simple act of becoming vegan, I believe, moves the soul or spirit or essence or energy or whatever you wish to call it, to wake up to a deeper affinity to all that lives. And we begin to feel from within our very core that "In the end, only kindness matters". It really is entirely impossible to feel the truth of this transformation without taking this first simple, deeply compassionate step. We can only ever feel the truth of this by allowing oneself to embrace this next stage in the evolution of the heart.

Let's face it, we find ourselves as vegans among some of the greatest people in human antiquity. We have the Buddha, Pythagoras, Ovid,

Saint Francis of Assisi, Leonardo Da Vinci, Voltaire, William Blake, Percy and Mary Shelley, just to name a few. For our times we have Philip Wollen (philanthropist, and animal activist), Peter Singer, AC, (author, moral philospher and profesor of Bioethics), James Cameron (film maker), Howard Lyman (author and activist), Dr. Will Tuttle (author, musician, speaker & educator), Gene Stone (author and ghost writer), Novak Djokovic (Tennis champion), Morgan Freeman (actor), Sia Furler (singer-songwriter, record producer), Moby (singer-songwriter), Joaquin Phoenix (actor, producer & animal activist), Bono of the band U2, Bryan Adams (singer-songwriter), Natalie Portman (actress), Brad Pitt (actor), Woody Harrelson (actor), Cameron Diaz (actress), Bill Clinton (Politician), Steve Jobs (inventor), Paul McCartney (musician and songwriter), Ellen DeGeneres (actress, comedian, and writer), David Murdock (businessman), Pamela Anderson (actress and model), Alicia Silverstone (actress), Stevie Wonder (singer-songwriter), Venus and Serena Williams (sports celebrities), Evanna Lynch (actress), Michelle Pfeiffer (actress), Jared Leto (singer and actor), Ariana Grande (singer and actress), Will.I.Am (singer-songwriter), and we see an increasing number of people worldwide all tuning to veganism. That gentle giant Patrik Baboumian is the world's strongest man who is of course also vegan. So we see filmmakers, actors, and actresses, writers, singers and people from all walks of life becoming vegan advocates.

It is indeed a very promising sign for the animals and the planet. Long may it go on growing, until the whole world embraces a new way of compassionate existence. And we enter a new age of love, compassion and kindness that will ultimately heal the world of all its abhorrent miseries. The only disclaimer I will add here is that sometimes people give up on veganism, and so I can confirm that at the time of writing, to the best of my knowledge, the people mentioned above were vegan. I should also add that we can never be totally certain of the historical figures I mention as being fully vegan, this is purely poetic licence on my part.

Doubts of Transition

"I am grateful to realize that my desires do not entitle me to add to another's suffering." Zoe Weil (1961–) co-founder and president of the Institute for Humane Education, author, and speaker.

I can still hear my own voice as a vegetarian saying: "Oh, I could never be vegan, because I love cheese too much". How many times have I heard that or similar from many, many other vegetarians? It was only after nearly dying from a severe asthma attack that I woke up to the simple fact that change was more than possible, especially if it meant putting my life on the line. Of course, just like all of our animal cousins, I did not want to die. In fact I rather liked being alive, as you probably do. I suspect that I am not alone in this desire to live out a full and healthy life as best I can. If this meant going vegan, well, I must confess I was ready to give it a try. The homoeopath I started consulting for my asthma suggested I read a book entitled *Fit for Life* by Harvey and Marilyn Diamond[1]. After reading it, I was determined to give it my best shot, and essentially became vegan almost overnight. I purchased a few vegan cookery books, including the classic Eva Batt's *Vegan Cooking*[2], which served me very well, and began the compassionate transformation of my eating habits, and I have to say, I have never once looked back. Food and cooking became a joy to me.

---

[1] www.amazon.com.au/Fit-Life-Harvey-Diamond/dp/0446553646

[2] www.amazon.com.au/Eva-Batts-Vegan-Cooking-Batt/dp/0722511612

This was in 1990, and at that time there were no premade vegan meals or products on the market. Thus, it was down to me to make all my meals from scratch. This is something that I still do to this day, and believe that this is the healthiest option for long term good health. One of the best parts of this transformation for me was that there was definitely and absolutely no vegan treats or cakes or cookies or anything of that nature available for me to buy, so I went sugar free. I did this by going 'cold turkey', but I am not convinced that this was the best path to take. I had a severe headache for about ten days straight! However, once it passed I was all-good! This is simply an example of detoxification. Once my gut flora adapted to the no sugar diet and found its equilibrium again, I was on a better path to good health. I remember once reading that the Chinese used to call sugar 'the white poison', it has also more recently been called the 'white death' by certain schools of thought.

The decision to become vegan was initially based on getting my health back on track, and to make progress in reducing my asthma symptoms. This was only one aspect of becoming vegan because once I joined the Vegan Society[3] founded by Donald Watson; I then knew where my path lay. I began to comprehend that as a global society, we had simply come to accept the atrocities of animal production as a cultural and necessary part of life. Yet, I also wondered were we perhaps simply all turning a 'blind eye' to the horrors of what brought food to our plate.

I realised very rapidly that there really was no logical, or emotional way back from becoming vegan. Not that I was looking for one. I also recognised that once we have taken this step, and we start to see the simple facts of the un-necessity of eating animals, which had always

---

[3] www.vegansociety.com

been horrifying to me, and their products, we change. We see that there is no room for a life where we live innocently in ignorance. I think for most of us transitioning from vegetarianism to veganism it is shocking to discover how blood bleeds so profusely from the dairy, and egg industries. Also, how the taking of honey leads to untold damage to the community and health of bees, alongside the horrors of the wool, leather and fur industries. Even to use the term 'industries' to describe what we do to our beautiful animal cousins is a euphemism at best, and an outrageously disgraceful lie at worst. Whatever anyone says, I cannot concede to this abominable trade in living beings, which is essentially slavery by another name.

Your Reason is Good Enough

"There is no fundamental difference between man and animals in their ability to feel pleasure and pain, happiness, and misery." Charles Darwin (1809–1882)

There is an important issue I would like to address here, and hopefully put an end to any debate on this dispute. It is the simple fact that it matters not, in any way, shape or form, how any individual becomes vegan. If anyone has the time to waste on such trivia, I would like to suggest that they might like to spend that invaluable time in the pursuit of something a little more productive. I feel that most vegans will probably never insult another person for making any attempt at living a more compassionate life. At least I would like to hope not. If we have good health, vigour and energy, then there is much that can be done that does not involve criticism of others. Whether or not you are a vegan activist, a vegan for good health, a vegan for the animals, a vegan for whatsoever reason, I salute and honour you, welcoming you into the wide world of compassion for all living beings. You are a hero in my eyes, and the world has precious little enough heroes.

It quite amazes me how the word 'terrorism' has ever been used by the media to describe vegans. If you take a cursory glance at any dictionary definition of this word, you would struggle to see how the word could be put in the same sentence as 'vegan'. The two words are as far apart in meaning as any two words can get, yet this is the game that the media plays with its audiences. Media is always about sensationalising whatever story they can, to make people sit up and take notice. And this all goes back to some of the early horrifying murder cases in Britain. Newspaper companies swiftly began to see that if they could fill the pages, especially the front headlines with something shockingly debauched, they would sell a lot more papers. Hence the saying: 'no news, is good news', which I appreciate has more than one meaning. The media can dress it up in whatever way they like. Yet it will never detract from the simple fact that vegans in whatever lifestyle they choose are by their very nature, endeavouring to put an end to the terrorism that billions upon billions of animals are living under. The real terrorism in this world is our treatment of animals. It also seems clear how the larger part of our global population has been blinded to the real facts of what goes on inside these insidious businesses.

The Oneness of Life

"Humankind has not woven the web of life. We are but one thread within it. Whatever we do to the web, we do to ourselves. All things are bound together. All things connect." Chief Seattle (1790–1866)

I believe that there is a beautiful oneness to being vegan in that it brings people together in unity of compassion. Of course, ultimately there is the Great Oneness that we are all part of, that is to say, that we are one with those we love, those we don't, in fact all and sundry, without a single exception. All the great spiritual traditions of the world have some form of story about this. Hinduism, and later Buddhism has the beautiful image of Indra's Net, which is a metaphor for the entire universe where each link in the net is a jewel of consciousness, a living sentient being, each linked together in the *Great Emptiness*. That is us, everyone, and of course, all our beautiful animal cousins. If we harm them, we ultimately harm ourselves.

There is no escape from this connection we all share, and that is why it is imperative that we realise one very important factor about our lives. Throwing hatred around does no one honour or justice, and it only serves to poison us from within. Hating the very thing that we wish to change can only ever block us to the universal creativity that is readily available when we let go of our anger. We want to see change, yes of course we do, and we want to stop the enslavement, the abuse, and the needless slaughter. Thus, it is through the joint gateway of love and compassion, which is the only way true and lasting change can take place in our world. The American writer Mark Twain, had something to say about this, he said: "Anger is an acid that can do more harm to the vessel in which it is stored than to anything on which it is poured", and I think this paints a clear picture about where our anger might actually take us; not I think, where we are really hoping to be.

Being Vegan is a Celebration of All Life

"... [T]he time will come when men such as I will look upon the murder of animals as they now look upon the murder of men." Leonardo da Vinci (1452–1519)

Being Vegan is a celebration of Life, *all life*, and really has absolutely nothing to do with self-deprivation or denial. Having said this, there is no harm in a little self-deprivation, for those of us living in the lap of luxury in the privileged world. The Quakers have a lovely saying about this: 'Live simply, so others may simply live'. If we want to help animals and all life on our beautiful planet, we must start at home within our own lives. I personally believe that physical health is a vitally important part of being vegan, so that we can go on helping for as long as possible and live by a beautiful and healthful example. There will always be exceptions to this general rule, and some people may well be held back by physical limitations, learning differences or even a debilitating illness, but I can say from personal experience that this does not always hold a person back, when they are in the grip of creativity and compassion. I am constantly amazed at the creative adaptation some people make to get things done and help this world of suffering, despite what would otherwise be seen as a potential impossibility. We could all learn something useful from the people that live under more challenging circumstances and still do great work.

All Round Good Health

"When people ask me why I don't eat meat or any other animal products, I say, 'Because they are unhealthy and they are the product of a violent and inhumane industry." Casey Afleck (1975–)

Positive mental health is essential if we really want to help the world. It is crucial to understand, as it has been suggested from the wise of the past, that if we hate others (for whatever self-justified reason), it is identical to drinking poison and thinking the other person is going to die. Ultimately, all we really achieve is suffering for ourselves, and nobody wants to suffer unnecessarily. It is important to note here that we don't need to suffer, just because the animals are suffering. We need a clear mind and a plan of action for the living of our lives in a compassionate way. If we feel true compassion for our cousins in the animal kingdom, then our lives should be a testament to finding a solution, and not to be bogged down in grief and despair at what we see and hear. If we really wish to make changes in the world we must be the example in every way possible, like the ancient Greek male citizens of the Polis who needed to be statesman, orator, poet, warrior and compassionate family man, all in one. We cannot and must not meet violence with violence - it can only end badly if we follow that path. To quote the political slogan by Jerry Garcia: "Constantly choosing the lesser of two evils is still choosing evil", and that is what we are endeavouring to get away from. We cannot create great change in this world of suffering, with evil intent. As the world's most notable scientist Einstein suggested in a letter to his daughter: *the power of love, on which the entire universe is based, will always win out. It is after all the greatest power we know.*

The Wonderful Power of Thought

"A man is but the product of his thoughts. What he thinks, he becomes."
Mahatma Gandhi (1869–1948)

The only way we can truly see the steps that are required in order to bring about great change is by understanding how our thinking creates our individual reality. If we remain in an angry state, we must recognise that this anger is coming from the way we are seeing things from our perspective, and ultimately our thinking about them. In other words, the anger is not coming from the violence we see enacted in the world against animals and other humans; that which we abhor. It is coming from our view of these circumstances. Anger and violence stems from thinking about the world, not from the world itself. Only when we see this clearly can we be set free to come up with the long-term solutions to these violent problems. As Zoe Weil, educator, writer and founder of the *Institute for Humane Education* suggests, we must become 'solutionaries' (a term I believe she coined). It is much, much harder to become a solutionary if we are down in the dumps in our spirits.

It is one thing to be informed about the abuses we wish to change and quite another to spend our time dwelling in the horror of it all. I would like to suggest that we really do have a choice here. I am not advocating a practice of denial, but moreover, a practice of calm, and meaningful action towards the end of this unnecessary barbarity. We can't choose the thoughts that enter our head, but we can choose which ones we give energy to, which ones we decide to focus on. And if we decide to keep thinking about all the pain and suffering in the world, we must expect to feel pretty low. Of course it is important to acknowledge that we can all feel low at times, and that is why it is so important to rest, recuperate and take care of ourselves in whatever way we can during these times. Love, compassion and companionship can also add great value during tough times.

It will be from a perspective of love and understanding that we make progress, not by reliving the horrors we know take place daily. Otherwise, all we do is keep drinking the proverbial poison of our own creation. Peace is a far superior force that will drive us to do great things in this world, with all its ups and downs and its violent sufferings. One of the greatest examples in history of non-violent activism is from Gandhi who inspired and led millions of people in a peaceful revolution to regain full independence for India back from the controlling forces of Britain. He may well not have been a perfect human being, as we all have our imperfections, so let us carry the message of hope that he created in millions, and use that as our baton of hope for the animals and the wild spaces of our planet. It is impossible to lead and inspire others to great deeds in peace if we hold anger and resentment in our hearts. We can only ever give away what and who we are. If we are only seen and portrayed by the media as an angry, subversive and aggressive group, we will fail to bring about the change we all desire. We must find new and creative ways to bring about the changes to which we all aspire, from all that we know to be wrong and harmful in the world.

One of the first questions most vegans get asked, besides the most exasperating: “where do you get your protein from?” (Which I will not deign to answer here, besides the fact that the question about protein is over a hundred years out of date), is “If you’re vegan, what on earth do you eat?” My answer to this bemusing question is: “Well, if you think of all the food in the world, all the edible plants and herbs, nuts, seeds, pulses, grains, fungi, fruits, and vegetables, vegans eat all of that, and only cut out dairy, honey, eggs, meats and fish”, essentially anything with eyes (with the exception of potatoes of course) or anything that comes from something with eyes. In other words, products produced from foods that are derived and ultimately stolen from animals.

One amusing story comes to mind here, many years ago while living in the UK, we were helping our neigbours with their hay harvest, and our hostess put on a big table in the garden a huge array of sumptuous foods for us to all enjoy after our hard days labour. One of the other helper’s teenage daughters heard some of us were vegan and said: “So what do vegans actually eat?” I just laughed in a good-humouredly manner, and said that literally everything that had been served up on the table was vegan! It is a strange thing indeed that people don't realise that most of what they eat on a daily basis is in fact vegan. The meal only becomes something other than vegan once the animal products are added.

One of the things I have always maintained since first becoming vegetarian in my teens is that far from missing 'things' that I had decided to no longer consume, I found I immediately embraced many the good foods that our beautiful planet had to offer. I would often wax lyrical about having enjoyed every single meal I had eaten since my departure from meat consumption. I could not say the same about the preceding years where I was forced to eat foods that made my stomach turn about in nauseating summersaults. I appreciate the simple fact that the majority of parents are doing the best they can, given the information they are 'fed' (no pun intended) about healthy eating. However, my poor father couldn't even eat in the same room as me for most meals, due to the fact of my struggle to eat what was literally vile to me, it probably made him gag as much as I did trying to swallow, what seemed to me as cannibalism.

I have to add here that my father didn't eat meat until he met and married my stepmother (who was an avid carnivore who thought the gristle was the best bit!), at the time I was still only a small boy, and my father's mother, our dear 'nana' didn't eat meat either, except in later years when her doctor innocently mislead her to believe she needed to eat some meat for protein! Oh, we are back to that old chestnut again, and so I would like to add a simple fact here about the composition of most fresh foods that a vegan might typically eat, they all contain some form of protein, even if it is in small amounts in some, and larger amounts in others, it is still there.

True protein deficiency is very rare especially in the modern western world, and I have never yet met a vegan diagnosed with a protein deficiency. Vitamin B-12 and Iron deficiency can become an issue for both vegans and vegetarians alike, and with a certain sense of irony, so too can meat eaters now become deficient in B-12 due to modern farming practices. These said modern farming practices lead directly to the animals themselves having this same deficiency. However, this is easily remedied for anyone being low in this vitamin, via naturally derived, ethically produced supplementation, which of course causes no suffering to animals in its production.

The vegan way of being is the start of living the good life. It is the evolution of the heart. The taking of an innocent life is never made spiritual by human ceremony; that is simply innocent superstition, ego, and sometimes bigotry. As a small child, one of my abiding memories was getting up early before the house was stirring and creeping downstairs, dragging most of my bedding with me to make a den out of the furniture in the lounge. Once this task was completed, it was into the pantry (kitchen food store) to get supplies. This often consisted of an immense chunk of Chocolate Swiss Roll deposited carefully into a bowl, into which I would push broken off pieces of digestive biscuits and smother this banquet of indulgence with lashings of cold milk. Then it was back to the hideout to feast on my provisions. Certainly not the healthiest breakfast in the world. As I have said, I was always a fussy child, and one of my other earliest memories was my mother threatening me with the need to eat 'bone broth' if I didn't eat what she gave me! So, it is clear that our personal relationship with food goes back to our earliest years, and food is often a source of comfort or discomfort to us, and therefore, it doesn't always feel easy to make the changes we may want to make.

However, if we wish to experience the transformation I spoke of earlier, we need to have the courage to make those changes first, and then we will see the benefits that flow from our new compassionate lifestyle of kindness. Having a diet based on love, not just our personal desire to satisfy our taste buds, is one that not only has a beautifying effect upon the world, as one removes oneself from becoming a living graveyard of our dead cousins, but also brings more peace and beauty within us. The peace that we desire, lies within us, it is already there at our core, and is simply made more beautiful and graceful when we stop putting pain and suffering on our plate, and then into our body.

Food is Life

"A man can live and be healthy without killing animals for food; therefore, if he eats meat, he participates in taking animal life merely for the sake of his appetite. And to act so is immoral." Leo Tolstoy (1828–1910)

It would seem to me that popular culture has the misguided notion that a vegan diet is somehow deficient, and it certainly is, it is deficient in cruelty, which I believe to be its greatest asset.

Food is life, but when it contains ingredients that have been forcibly taken from animals and ultimately leads to their destruction, it cannot be good for us and it cannot be good for the planet or for world peace. Where is peace in a placid cow only afforded a limited time to graze before being taken to slaughter? Where is peace in male baby chicks being killed as they will never make the cut as laying hens do? Most people never make the connection between what they eat and a deep sense of personal peace. That is of course, where world peace begins, within the hearts and minds of us all, the very people who populate this world. How can we expect peace to exist out there in the world if we continue to accept the needless slaughter of two billion sentient beings every week? Yes, you read that correctly *every week!* Most people who are tackled on this issue usually suggest that they themselves don't actually eat that much meat. However, the point is that when we calculate all of the demands for meat and dairy and fish in the world today, we accept the Frankenstenian monster of globalised factory based killing machines. We are either part of the solution or we are part of the problem, however small that part may be. Ultimately we must make that choice.

I remember once walking along a footpath out in the English countryside, in the beautiful County of Suffolk, with my partner at the time. This was several years after becoming vegan, probably about 1996. It was a beautiful summer's day and I noticed some cows in a field, and as I stopped to gaze at them grazing, they got curious and came to say hello. I was so moved by their majestic beauty and their wonderfully inquisitive nature that I was moved to tears, knowing where they would ultimately end up. I gave my pitifully inadequate apologies to these amazing beings and moved on with a heavy heart. I have never really been able to reconcile in myself how we as beings can eat such beauty. If it were up to me, I mused, this would all end, then, now, and forever.

The Shape of Things to Eat

"Healthy eating is a way of life, so it's important to establish routines that are simple, realistically, and ultimately livable." Quintus Horatius Flaccus, otherwise known as Horace (65–8 BCE)

I find this topic profoundly fascinating and believe that it is worth mentioning here; that is to say that vegans are often criticised for eating 'mock meats'. Now, I must say I am not really a fan of anything that looks or tastes like meat, and I am not all that big on processed foods either. There is much debate about how good processed foods are for health. These faux meats also trigger in me some pretty unpleasant memories of what I was once forced to eat, and I must add, this was very much against my personal will. However, as mentioned earlier in the book, there are many paths that lead a person to becoming vegan, and I for one, don't have a problem with any of them. There is a huge and growing industry, singularly intent on producing 'mock meat' and vegan alternatives to the growing demand from an ever-increasing vegan public. This is how all markets work, if there is a demand for something, there will be a growth pattern and companies will literally trip over each other to fill the market with the desired end products that are in demand.

From one perspective, this is a wonderful sign indeed, because it points very directly towards the fact that a lot more people are moving away from meat consumption, and that is a great place to start towards a better world. If there was no demand, there would be no products, and any attempt at producing such products would be deemed to fail. But there is something else here that is also intriguing in the criticisms aimed at vegans, and it is this: why do vegans want to eat things that look, but maybe don't actually taste like meat products, if they don't like meat? i.e., a sausage, a burger etc. Well, to start with, some vegans do actually like meat, but they have made the decision to become vegan, because it is to them an issue of ethics, not taste or shape. My argument is always that these are simply nouns; they name the shape of the food, and do not denote the contents of the food itself, that is innocently assumed. So, people may assume that a sausage is made of meat, but it can just as easily be a vegan sausage, or burger or mince. Or it could be a dairy substitute made with coconut oil, such as yoghurt or cheese, or a milk alternative. It is to my mind a very strange criticism, and yet another part of the total misunderstanding of someone who has made the choice to become vegan. I hardly think it worth the effort and lengths that some people seem to go to criticise and demean a person for deciding to live a more ethical life. However, the hero is often debased, and ironically, by those who stand on very unsound ethical ground. To criticise ethical behaviour seems to me a very strange thing to do. Having said this, again I would suggest that criticism is done in innocence, for each one of us is doing the best we can, given our in the moment thinking.

Human Induced Enviromental Devastation

"By eating meat we share the responsibility of climate change, the destruction of our forests, and the poisoning of our air and water. The simple act of becoming a vegetarian will make a difference in the health of our planet." Thich Nhat Hanh (1926–2022)

There is absolutely no doubt that animal agriculture is causing a massive increase in land and water based pollution and virgin deforestation. Additionlly, there is huge increase in methan gas production from animal agriculture which is reputed to be a significant element of the drastic climate changes we are seeing in the world today. Kip Andersen, the maker of *Cowspiracy* the documentary, was totally perplexed why almost all of the environmental agencies he contacted during the making of the documentary could not, or would not answer the simple question: 'What is the number one cause of climate change?' This is at present a serious and contentious issue, which I do not claim to be qualified to write about. However, what does seem apparent is the rapidly increasing frequency of enviromental catastrophies.

Not taking positive action in the face of the overwhelming evidence that animal production is one of the main causes of human induced environmental descruction is tantamount to global suicide. Personally, I don't believe everyone wants to take their own life; in fact I know the opposite to be true. Everyone alive wants to live a good life and is trying to get there; doing the best they can to achieve that. What I also believe is that even those poor souls that are on the brink of suicide, are just like us, they just want the suffering they are experiencing to go away, and to have that good life that seems so elusive to them, and I imagine that the last dramatic and fatal act is that attempt to find the peace we all desire by putting an end to the misery of their lives. Just like Tolstoy's ill fated 'Anna Karenina' in her last moment of consciousness realises too late that she really wants to live. I will add that on those occasions when I begin to feel overwhelmed with aspects of my life and what I perceive to be a lack of time, I endeavour to keep the following words in mind:

"Don't say you don't have enough time. You have exactly the same number of hours per day that were given to Helen Keller, Pasteur, Michelangelo, Mother Teresa, Leonardo da Vinci, Thomas Jefferson, and Albert Einstein." H. Jackson Brown Jr. (1940–)

A lone calf under a tree

"The greatness of a nation and its moral progress can be judged by the way its animals are treated." Mahatma Gandhi (1869-1948)

While on a canoeing trip with one of my daughters in the Riverina, in Western New South Wales, Australia, I was driving along an irrigation channel and I spotted a small calf under a tree, standing as still as a statue. This is a common sight on hot days in the dry western part of NSW; however, there was something wrong with this particular image. It reminded me of a story I was once told by a local farmer while I was working in this part of the country. He said that when he needed to move cattle from one field to another for better water in the dry, if cattle could smell the water nearby they would give him hell and keep running back towards the water in a more direct route, and he would have a hard job getting them through the gate, as they would constantly move towards the shortest route to it, despite there being a barbed wire fence in the way to get there, and no gate in that spot.

One of the other behaviours dairy cows have, is when the farmer decides that it is time to separate them from their calves, a mother would hide her baby in among scrub and bush and communicate to the little one that it was not to move until she the mother returns. This farmer assured me that the calf would simply stay hidden and motionless indefinitely and wait for the mother to return, and even die if she did not come back. The farmer said that you could spend days trying to locate these hidden young and the mothers would always be trying to get back to them. This poor calf I witnessed standing motionless under the tree a long way from the sight of any other animals may well have been one of these so instructed young, waiting in hope for his mother to return. If you have any doubt about the intelligence of cows or their deep family connections please read Rosamund Young's *The Secret Life of Cows*[4].

The Lost Lamb

"Animal factories are one more sign of the extent to which our technological capacities have advanced faster than our ethics." Peter Singer (1946–)

Not dissimilarly, I remember being on a solitary camping trip in Wales, in the UK and on the first night of the trip there was a terrible

[4] www.amazon.com.au/Secret-Life-Cows-Rosamund-Young/dp/0525557318

commotion. The place I was camping in was on a farm, and they had just moved their flock of sheep and newly born lambs into a new field. It would seem that one poor little creature had managed to either get left behind or somehow got through a tiny gap in the hedgerow and become separated from its mother. All night long the unfortunate lamb piteously cried out in the dark and ran frantically up and down the field to the bellowing calls of its mother from the other side of the hedge, until they were reunited again the following day when the farmer came to check how they all were. Of course the poor mother and her calf would have to go through this same trauma again when the farm carried out its barbaric practice of separation from mother, and segregation of male and female for high productivity and profit. This is simply slavery of a different kind, this time not through colour of skin, but simply through the innocent blindness of speciesism.

Another story I was told more recently by an ex-dairy and beef cattle farmer (turned close to vegan) where they described how the thing that drove them to give up on the trade was the job of taking the cattle to slaughter. Initially, he described that when he needed to separate the mother cows from their young in order to wean them to prepare them either for the veal industry or to fatten them for the beef and leather industry. As mentioned in the story above the mothers would sense what was happening and take their young as far away as possible in order to prevent separation.

Fear of Death

"All beings tremble before violence. All fear death, all love life. See yourself in others. Then whom can you hurt? What harm can you do?" Guatama Siddhartha (lived at the latter part of the first millennium BCE)

This same ex-farmer went on to recount how when taking his cattle to the slaughterhouse, at least a kilometre out from the hideous destination, the cows would start a terrible commotion within the back of the truck. They would invariably go wild and start kicking and pushing, and hustle and shove and begin an unearthly screaming for this final part of the journey; some he insisted would do everything to get out of the truck while it was still moving. He said it would happen every single time without fail and not a living soul could convince him that they didn't know what was coming next. He told me how he simply couldn't go on in the same way, and couldn't bear to see the suffering these beautiful creatures were going through. I think that there is a myth in most cultures that humans have the unfortunate ability to know that one day, they are going to die, and that animals have escaped this misery of knowledge. However, I think this story illustrates that animals may not have foresight about the coming of death, but when it is close and impending doom awaits them, they most certainly want to avoid it in the same way as humans would. Especially if humans were loaded onto trucks in large numbers and in cramped conditions, and then began to smell the blood in the air and begin to feel the fear of what would become their fate.

From an ethical perspective, consuming the flesh of another species in order to sustain our own skin is a cruel and selfish act, and the consequences on our lives can carry a very heavy weight. Having said this, there is a huge dichotomy between a person purchasing meat to cosume, and the killing of the animal. As in most cases, people don't usually take part in the killing, and so are removed and dissasociated from its violence. This ultimately leads to *Cognitive Dissonance.* As mentioned before, peace has to begin with the individual, not something out there in the world. The late Buddhist author and founder of the Western Buddhist Order, Sangharakshita suggests in a book of the same title that: *Peace is a Fire*, not, as many may assume, that peace is a form of passivity, but moreover it is an act of authority against injustice everywhere. From one small action of kindness grows an enormous mountain of goodwill, love and compassion that runs around the world like a bushfire in high winds. It is like throwing a pebble in a pond and the ripples have an everlasting positive outcome down through time. This is what we are part of when we make the decision to become vegan, and live an ethical life. It is a powerful act of defiance against a corrupt, unethical and outdated mode of living in the world.

I have had it on good account from a number of ageing farmers, that the older they get the harder it becomes for them to send their animals to slaughter. Their reflections seem to be mainly based around the idea of their own inevitable demise, a thing we must all face one day. Yet, the idea of sending what amounts to be very young animals to their doom, long before they have had a chance to live out a full and healthy life as we all hope to do. I say ageing farmers, but I must confess that this is not strictly true, as I am now meeting more and more younger people who have grown up around animals and are finding it increasingly difficult to send our beautiful cousins to their untimely end. Awareness, it would seem, is growing and people are returning to a more natural sense of compassionate ethics. Long may this last, and swift may be its progress.

Change in History

"The secret of change is to focus all of your energy, not on fighting the old, but on building the new." Dan Millman (1946–)

An example of this from the history of great change, is that of William Wilberforce (1759 – 1833), not only did he spend a large part of his life fighting the slave trade, which was no small task at the time, but he was also the founder of the RSPCA (Royal Society for the Protection of Animals), and worked tirelessly for plight of animals and their suffering. As Stephen Tompkins clearly explains: 'When Wilberforce stood before parliament to propose the abolition of the slave trade … the number of people in comparable forms of forced labour throughout the world was something like 75 per cent. Today is one-fifth of 1 per cent.'[5] The exciting thing about this example is that despite opposition of an unprecedented nature, which stood in his way, and the many others, that worked alongside Wilberforce in his endeavours to secure freedom for the slaves, its effects can still be seen in the world today. This should give us all great hope for the plight of animals the world over. It is now our turn to take up the baton of what began almost three hundred years ago and make it stronger, better and larger than ever before. And as mentioned earlier, our most important and vital ally in this great work is our personal mental wellbeing and mindset. If this is strong, then our resolution to bring about big change is more than possible. We are most definitely up against an equally powerful adversary as our forerunners were, if not a greater force; yet we have the history of great achievements on our side, and with international ecommerce and the Internet, we have a very formidable partner to move towards big and lasting change.

---

[5] William Wilberforce: A Biography, Stephen Tomkins, William B. Eerdmans Publishing Company, Grand Rapids, Michigan/Cambridge U.K.

Vevolution

"Non-violence leads to the highest ethics, which is the goal of all evolution. Until we stop harming all other living beings, we are still savages."
Thomas Edison (1847–1931)

A good friend of mine, a professor in Philosophy, has a wonderful way of ending any potential arguments about either being vegetarian or vegan. When people demand a justification for such an act, he would simply answer: "It is perfectly simple my dear friend, it is evolution." Thus, we are either evolving towards a compassionate way of living or we are stuck. Stuck, as it were with tradition, culture, the status quo, convention, the way things have always been done. But it doesn't have to be that way. And what a beautiful part of evolution to be at; to be consciously aware that what we do in the name of some outdated tradition or whatever it might be, can be put down, left behind and we can move forward with more kindness, more compassion, and more love for all life on earth. Not just human life, or the few animals we see as pets, and not food but all sentient life. It is what some are calling *vevolution*.

It is impossible to force evolution on anyone, any more than our ancestors could on the Neanderthals. It is important to recognise that this is evolution and not revolution: Evolution is the natural path from living one way and then adapting to living and thriving in a new way. Whereas revolution usually requires violence and force to bring about change that the world and its status quo is firmly and violently opposed to. As Philip Wollen has reminded us many times, the man of peaceful action Mahatma Gandhi posited that when one is presenting a seemingly radical idea to the world, firstly it is ignored, then ridiculed, then it is forcibly resisted, and then it is accepted. In other words, we could potentially force people to stop eating meat and animal products via politics and law. That is, should there be such a will in those in power, (yet I feel that is highly unlikely to happen) nevertheless, we cannot make people become vegan. To become a vegan is a choice that leads to a beautiful transformation from within, that has enormous consequences and benefits to the outside world. Of course, people giving up meat and dairy would be a great place to start, as I believe this would, in most circumstances, lead to more compassionate awareness. As my dear friend the late Dr. Roger Mills once put it: "people don't change because they feel they are wrong, people change because they have a personal insight about the way they are living", and from this insight, they decide to make ethical changes in their lives. Everyone alive has the same potential for personal change; all we need to do is look within, to our common sense and wisdom, to see that the ethical life is the best life to live. And living this way is certain to bring about a deeper sense of peace within.

Begin at the beginning

"The vegan diet is healthy and leads to a compassionate lifestyle. I've gotten so many benefits. My weight is easily maintained, my skin glows, I sleep better and I feel more energized." Meagan Duhamel (1985–)

Here is a short and gentle guide for those wishing to live in a non-violent way for the good of all life:

Compassion towards all living beings includes oneself. Thus, any act of self-abuse such as drugs, alcohol, tobacco, a poor diet, or self-inflicted sleep deprivation, all point towards lack of self love and respect for oneself. This too is a form of innocently activated violence. Should one wish to argue that working long and arduous hours for the animals is essential to bring about this change, I believe that we can all be so much more effective in our endeavours to help the animals if we eat well, sleep well and always give ourselves the time to rest, rejuvenate and revitalise. There may well be times when extra effort for a selected time period may be of great benefit, but to make this the rule, as it were, will ultimately lead to us being less effective, and may even lead to sickness. This applies to not only our body, but our inimitable spirit also. As Stephen Covey suggests in his classic book *The Seven Habits of Highly Effective People*[6]: "We need to sharpen the saw", in other words give over time to do the things we love in order to become sharper once back in the driving seat of our lives. Then we can return with renewed vigour, energy and greater creativity, to guide us on the path to bring about great and lasting change.

If we allow ourselves to break free from the bonds of this world and let our spirit soar, we will inevitably rise to ever-greater heights of compassion for all life. The creativity we need to solve the problems we face arises out of a quiet mind, not from a full mind. As Einstein once suggested: '... Imagination is more important than knowledge. Knowledge is limited. Imagination encircles the world'[7]. And I think you will agree, we need a solution for the animals that will 'encircle the [whole] world.' Additionally, it is always worth remembering that moments of wisdom, clarity and insight can occur at any second, and so often come about when we are least expecting them to, this is because they arise within a timeless zone. Einstein once suggested

---

[6] www.amazon.com.au/Habits-Highly-Effective-People-Anniversary/dp/1760856827

[7] www.saturdayeveningpost.com/2010/03/imagination-important-knowledge/

that all of his greatest scientific discoveries came about when he was walking his dog in the park daydreaming.

To be in the World, but not of it

"The reasonable [hu]*man adapts himself to the world; the unreasonable one persists in trying to adapt the world to himself. Therefore all progress depends on the unreasonable man."* George Bernard Shaw (1856–1950)

To use the well-known Christian phrase, 'to be in the world but not of the world' serves us well here. We can never simply be victims of our circumstances, either past or present; we can only ever be victims of the way we think about these circumstances and the world at large. In any given moment we can rise up from the most deplorable surroundings and circumstances and move forward to live an ethical and compassionate life. The choice is ours to make, if we can but see that we create our reality via our own personal thinking. I have watched with amazement how some people, despite their physical limitations, can and do make immense efforts for the good of animals. Conditions that would floor, if not at least stall most people, are simply overcome via a boundless strength of mind, and incredible adaptations to their lives to make things work. It is truly amazing to see what can be achieved with a quiet and still mind. This will ever humble me, having been witness to its magic.

The animals have no voice, at least not one that we can as yet fully understand. Although, having said this, we each have the innate ability to communicate our love and compassion towards animals, and all life forms on earth, just as we do for our loved ones. I have certainly met people that have a captivating way of communicating with animals, which is a beautiful thing to witness. Regardless, we can be certain that animals do not give their consent to us, to take from them what is rightful for their offspring, and ultimately take the gift of their life from them. What I am suggesting here is for our voice to become a unanimous voice of protest against the so-called industries that enslave, torture, mutilate and slaughter with impunity. We must become the voice for the voiceless.

Drugs and Alcohol

"Relax, allow the mind to become empty, and surprise yourself with the great treasure that begins to flow from your soul." Paulo Coelho. (1947–)

A few words about drugs and alcohol: firstly there is no such thing as commercially produced purely vegan alcoholic drinks that I am aware of. This is due to the fact that all non-organic plant production involves chemical based fertilisers, herbicides, pesticides and fungicides, all of which kill millions of insects, which in turn get consumed by birds, small mammals, lizards and frogs, forcing its way up the food chain as one species eats another. If we take wine as a simple example on its own, when the grapes are mechanically harvested and get transported to the press for the first part of its production, the grapes going into the press contain insects, spiders, ants, lizards, snakes, and sometimes even frogs. Thus there are body parts and blood right at the start. So, even if we put aside the issue of fish blood or dairy derived finings used in most conventional wine production to make the wine clear, we are still left with the problem of all of those lovely creatures that went into the press. This is not to say of course, that organic production is all that much different when it comes to producing alcohol, because the same creatures will still be present on organically grown vines too.

As for drugs and tobacco products, it becomes clear that production of these substances are going to cause harm almost all the way along the chain of production and manufacture. Not to mention the horrendous end results as families lose loved ones to a life of drugs, and the inevitable insidious and multiple forms of tobacco induced cancer and other diseases. If we wish to live in harmony with the planet and at peace with all living beings we must do our best to put aside these so-called 'addictions' and live a cleaner, healthier, happier and more productive life – just as nature intended. When we do this, we are repaid in kind by nature itself.

The Joy of Being Alive

"If having a soul means being able to feel love and loyalty and gratitude, then animals are better off than a lot of humans."
James Herriot (1916–1995)

Looking again at the cattle industry, before farmers castrate young males, a vile and barbaric practice, I have often witnessed how, when herded together, these young creatures will run and jump and cavort, kicking their legs high into the air, as they play in the utter joy of being alive, and not forgetting the sheer delight of being together. Indeed, most animals in the wild have been witnessed to do likewise. This can be said the same for lambs and probably all of the young of our so-called domesticated animals that we so unfittingly call 'livestock'. I can remember many occasions where I have personally witnessed large numbers of lambs finding a raised spot or hillock in a field, and each in turn taking a run at the spot and jumping off as if on spring loaded legs, a true joy to behold. It is as if we can reduce the life of a beautiful creature to nothing more than a stock item to be used and abused as though it were an inanimate object of little or no consequence, and without the feeling and emotions that we experience. If this is not enough for us to see the consciousness and awareness of these beautiful creatures then we have become blind to the true beauty of this world, because there is nothing of beauty in the taking of a life. Killing with compassion is one of the biggest lies of the animal agricultural industries. This is hypocrisy at its highest level, and I reject it with every fibre of my being.

A friend in Hawaii once told the story of an incident that occurred with one of her husband's cows. The cow's little calf had been sick, and while the couple were out having a meal, they received a call from their neighbour, who had been keeping an eye on the place to let them know that one of the cows was making a lot of noise and they should check it out when they got home. Previously there had been a big storm and the calf had become sick and the mother would not leave its side, attempting to keep it warm and cleaning it. After a while all of the other cows in the herd gathered round the mother and calf.

What had transpired while the couple were out at dinner was that the calf had died and the mother was lamenting its death with the most unusual and frightening sounds. The mother went on calling out all night long. The next day they dug a pit and buried the calf, but the mother would not leave the burial site and continued calling out in a harrowing, distressed way. All the other cattle stayed gathered around the mother and they even attempted to move the earth from the buried calf. How much evidence does any one need to see the obvious and striking notion that animals, just like us, have feelings and emotions and create bonds with each other and their young. There is an old saying that goes something like this: "There is a good reason why we take our children to the hobby farm, and *not* to the slaughterhouse". I can only imagine an entire generation of very youthful vegans, if parents decided to do the latter. How could we expect a child to ever want to eat meat again, if they at once realised that the very animals they just petted and cuddled were now sliced up on their plate ready to eat! I feel this would not be very likely. It is this dichotomy and lie by which our society is duped as these industries continue to carry out their barbaric practices behind very closed doors, and hidden from the world.

Slaughter of the Innocent

"As long as there are slaughterhouses there will always be battlefields."
Leo Tolstoy (1828–1910)

It is said that people who work in the slaughter industry only last a few short years before they start to suffer psychologically, and need to move on and get out. I must say that I am surprised that they last that long. I don't think that fact is at all surprising to anyone, given that it is such an unnatural thing to do, to take life in cold blood, almost like a psychopathic murderer. To do this on a daily basis for work, is neither natural nor ethical to ask this of a human being. It is to a large extent knowingly dehumanising the individual, which will have the inevitable consequences of affecting their family directly and society perhaps more indirectly. Neither of which can ever really serve a good purpose. I believe that while we continue to run our enormous killing machines, true and lasting peace for global society will continue to elude us as a species, as mentioned before we live in an almost constant state of *Cognitive Dissonance*. People are often heard speaking of their love of animals, and yet consciously don't seem to make the connection between loving some animals, and eating others, therein lies the contradiction of our discordant beliefs. If we wish to put an end to this state of affairs, then the more people can be educated to the facts of what we do to animals the better. There are many active vegan groups around the globe that do such educational work in their spare time, and this I cannot praise highly enough. What great and worthy work this is.

In terms of health it is neither necessary nor essential for humans to eat meat[8] or animal products for good, vibrant and lasting health. Therefore, one can only assume that individuals innocently use their own free will to partake in the end result of an act of violence against other species to satisfy a want and their taste buds. In doing so they deny the free will of animals to live out a free and natural life in peace. With the education programs mentioned above, peace begins to spread its wings among the general population, and people once educated, cannot simply live in ignorance any longer. This is a source of great hope for the animals.

Cut off in their prime as animals so often are, it would seem that those that trade in our living beautiful cousins, begin to feel the suffering and untimely death of those that they have been playing guardian for. As previously stated, our connection to animals is of a different order than with each other. When we fully recognise this connection and begin to feel it, we must honour this understanding. I imagine it would be almost impossible to continue to condemn to death those we have tenderness for. Life it would seem has a way of teaching us a deeper compassion, even if we are not looking for it. Love, as I have repeated in this book, being the greatest force in the Universe, eventually has its way of instructing us to live a better life.

---

[8] According to Phillip Wollen, and Ivy League Universities Cornell and Harvard: 'the optimum amount of meat in a healthy diet is precisely Zero. Thus, the argument that meat consumption is an essential part of a healthy diet is simply a myth.

Speciesism

"We will, at some point, reflect back at our rampant acceptance of speciesism with profound regret. Our journey to understanding that all demonstrations of life possess equal value is a slow and harrowing one."
Ian Somerhalder (1978–)

Have we not been told since birth (and I imagine this is part of most cultures), that we should not steal from others? Yet, here we are living in a largely global society that happily and purposefully 'takes the not given' (to use the Buddhist term for this) from animals. Which is purely and simply stealing. It has to be, by its very nature, because we do not ask the animals if they mind if we take their milk, their honey, their wool, their body to be eaten, and their skin to be made into clothes. We do not ask them because we do not believe they share an experience of living consciousness as we do. It would seem that some people see these precious animals as nothing more than objects to be used and abused as they see fit. But, however we dress this up, reword or re-imagine it, it is stealing. Thus we often live by a vastly disproportionate double standard of our societies' making. Society and industry innocently uses speciesism as its benchmark to differentiate between human animals and non-human animals, yet it is obvious if looked at rationally that we and the animals are in fact one. There is no separation between us, only the separation we create via our own thinking for the simple convenience of continuing these same barbaric and outdated practices. We dress it up in the lies of commerce, culture, tradition, folklore, myth, ritual, legend and belief to make opposites out of a mirroring.

What is fascinating about this is that most bright healthy people don't practice bigotry, racism, sexism, chauvinism, or any other form of discrimination, but it seems that many a good person will innocently and actively practice speciesism. Almost every time these same people go shopping or prepare a meal for their loved ones they unwittingly enact speciesism. The question is often asked: why do we love dogs and cats and a litany of other 'domesticated' animals yet we are happy to slaughter and eat others? What is this, if not a violent and cruel form of speciesism? As Dr. Albert Schweitzer once suggested: 'The thinking [hum]man must oppose all cruel customs no matter how deeply rooted in tradition or surrounded by a halo ... We need a boundless ethic which will include the animals also'.[9]

As mentioned above, we cannot truly say we love animals (as many people claim to do) and then eat them or take their milk from them and kill their young at the same time. There is a gulf here of enormous proportions that people are ignoring or suppressing within themselves; and we do this in order to satisfy an unnecessary want in ourselves. Peace must, and always will begin within the very depths of our own soul, spirit, essence, energy or whatever you want to call it. We cannot take life and call it by any other name than what it is: *murder*. Life is the greatest gift we are given, why should any being be denied its right to live out a full and healthy existence here in paradise.

For the Want of Food

"Hunger is not a problem. It is an obscenity. How wonderful it is that nobody need wait a single moment before starting to improve the world."
Anne Frank (1929–1945)

---

[9] Cited in 'Testing times in toxicology-In Vitro vs In Vivo Testing', https://proceedings.altex.org/data/2013-01/rISC_008_Pereira1.pdf

There is a direct correlation between people starving in developing countries and animal production, this may only be one part of this complex system but it is yet another layer of violence that we innocently give our support and encouragement to when we consume flesh and animal products of every kind. One of the factors involved in this is that we feed grain and pulses to animals, that they have not evolved to eat, in huge feedlots and 'factory farms' (I can think of a better term), in order to keep the meat rolling out in a cheap as chips form, while men, women and children starve to death in some of the same countries where the crops are grown. It is sometimes hard to believe that there are more cattle on planet earth today than there are people; there is something seriously wrong with this equation. Concerningly, much of the land used to grow these crops is either native forest, stripped bare, or filled with animals that are tagged for future slaughter and put out to pasture on this land. Inevitably after a few short years the land simply dries up and the topsoil blows away, rendering the land useless and purposeless for anything at all. One of the solutions to this problem lies in the field of agroforestory and permaculture, something the indigenous peoples of the world have been practicing for thousands of years.

Understanding this gives us the opportunity to make careful decisions about where our food comes from. That we can make healthy and ethical decisions about what we consume, with our prior knowledge about its sources. Of course, many people are now returning to the natural tradition of growing their own food at home in the garden, as my generations' grandparents did. I am not suggesting that vegans should, or must be fit and live healthily, but I am posing the question, why wouldn't you want to be fit and healthy? It is unquestionable that research supports the fact that vegans often have a longer duration of life. I question you, is the ability to live a longer, healthier and more fulfilling life something that you would like? If we love life and want to help animals, surely it would be better to have good energy, fitness and health to primarily do more good in the world for animals. And secondly prove, through our living a good life that it is more than adequate to live as a vegan, and in fact to show the simple fact that vegans thrive living as they do. Is this not reason enough and a beautiful thing to show to the world? Rather than, to borrow the phrase from Joe Cross' documentary, *Fat, sick and nearly dead*, as so much of the world population is today. Obesity is a lifestyle disease, and not only completely reversible, but moreover, easily preventable via a wholefoods plant based vegan diet. A standard western diet, to put it bluntly, is a big killer. As the Lancet suggested in a 2019 paper[10]: 'Unhealthy diets pose a greater risk to morbidity and mortality than does unsafe sex, and alcohol, drug, and tobacco use combined.' That's a really big statement right there, and something definitely worth contemplating.

Animal Experimentation

"We know we cannot be kind to animals until we stop exploiting them — exploiting animals in the name of science, exploiting animals in the name of sport, exploiting animals in the name of fashion, and yes, exploiting animals in the name of food." César Chávez (1927–1993)

It is important to remember that people not only eat animals and their products, but in the name of science, they torture, mutilate and ultimately destroy and discard what is no longer useful to them via the dubious term 'vivisection'. All this is carried out supposedly to

[10] www.thelancet.com/journals/lancet/article/PIIS0140-6736(18)31788-4/fulltext

help the human race remain healthy and not to be unnecessarily exposed to dangerous chemicals, products, foods and medicines. While we take these potentially harmful products and foods and pour them into eyes, douse exposed skin, and inject them into various, so called 'farmed animals', and wild animals stolen from nature. I am not sure I can fully comprehend, not only how a human being could do such cold blooded and callous 'work', but also how they can continue to do this day in day out. It is a wonder to me how society manages to hold it together at all, given the barbarity of what we do in the name of science and food. We are, I believe, as a global society so totally immersed in what I am calling *annibalism*, that most people, simply don't want to acknowledge this horror and consternation, and as a result proceed with the fantastical beliefs that many animals are living joyous lives in their perfectly kept farms, with their ultimate death being quite natural and of course humane. If that is not a contradiction in terms, I have no idea what is. How does one take the life of an innocent being, and conduct this barbarity humanely? I don't believe it can be done; it is just another lie to go with general fabrication of deceit that has been created to prevent ordinary people asking obvious questions. And these are questions that must be asked; why do we keep doing this?

If we use make-up and hair colourants, wear deodorant, take medications and accept vaccinations without question, we innocently add to the mass suffering of animals. This can be partially overcome through researching what are the most ethical and non-harmful products available. We have a choice here that society does not have the right to refuse us. We can freely choose which companies we will support, which banks we keep our money in, what food products we purchase and consume. As mentioned before, it is almost impossible to be totally ethical, because we live in a largely uncaring, unethical corporate economy, which places profit far above ethical behaviour towards animals, compassion and a care for the environment and our dwindling wild places. Yet, we can do our very best in what, how and where we purchase the necessities of life, becoming as ethical as it is possible to be. One only has to do a brief Internet search to discover recipes and instructions on how to make self-care and health care products at home, and many of the things we now see as essential to life. Various household cleaning products, deodorants, skin care products and many other things can be made of safe and healthy ingredients, costing very little and from within the comfort of our own homes.

I remember once many years ago, lying on the grass in a park on a sunny day, daydreaming. In my imagination I saw a small monkey clinging to a tree licking the dewdrops from a leaf, his hair damp from the morning mist. His mother has been taken, there was no milk for his hungry belly, so he must eat what he can to survive; for his mother will not return from the lab she has been taken to. A tear forms in his eyes, almost too small for our eyes to see. Missing the embrace and warmth of a mother's touch he clings helplessly from the tree of my dreams. If only I could save him and all his kind, I might feel I had been of some use in this world of torture of the innocent.

I am certain that I am not alone in having such musings and desires, let us all hope we can put a permanent end to these barbaric practices.

Domestic Pets and other creature comforts

"Any glimpse into the life of an animal quickens our own and makes it so much larger and better in every way." Johh Muir (1838-1914)

It is worth taking a brief look at the notion of keeping animals as pets. I fully appreciate the comfort they bring many people, and I have very fond memories of our family's pet dog Toby who lived until he was seventeen. I have to say just how deeply heartbroken I was when he died. I realised at that moment, that our connection to animals and more importantly, our relationship with them is profound, and it somehow goes beyond the loss we may feel when we lose a human family member. Perhaps this is to do with the totally non-verbal relationship we share with them, and so the emotional feelings run deeper. Animals inherently understand unconditional love. I wept for a long, long time, while my brother (on the other end of the phone) did his best to console me, he, I knew, was feeling it too. That feeling of loss stayed with me for some time, and other friends have shared similar stories of this kind, you too may have your own.

However, there is a darker side to this comfort we feel in having pets. I am glad to say that there are many new vegan friendly pet foods around, which takes part of the sting out of owning pets. I also appreciate that many vegans and non-vegans take in rescue dogs, cats, chickens, and ducks etc. In fact even larger animals are rescued and taken to our many wonderful animal sanctuaries. But the question remains, where do all these lost creatures come from, especially the dogs and cats? Unfortunately, most come from puppy farms, pet shops and the like. While we have such an industry, we will always have strays, abused and neglected animals that need a good home, and they don't all make it. Many are euthanized because they are deemed as having been around for too long, and the shelters simply cannot afford to keep them any longer. It is a difficult and contentious subject and I am not suggesting that I have the answers, just that these issues need addressing.

The darkest aspect to our pet loving is what pets most often are fed. I have met vegans that feed their pets minced meat, arguing that this is the most natural diet for a cat or dog. However, primarily all we are doing is playing into the hands of the globalised killing machines as we feed our pets, the waste products of this industry. The parts that humans mostly don't like to consume. I am not suggesting for one moment that anyone should do this, but if we were to look at what is most natural for a cat to eat, then we would need to start finding rats, mice, lizards, frogs and small birds. For this would be more natural than unwanted parts of a cow, pig, sheep, horse or goat. When was the last time you saw a domestic cat stalking any of these larger ruminants? It would be too laughable to contemplate, were it not so sad. How can we practise compassion by not eating animals and animal products, if we then feed them to our pets? Then we are condoning the killing of a certain number of species in order to feed the ones we call pets. It just doesn't make any ethical sense.

I have also heard it argued that vegan pet food is unnatural and unfair to feed to animals that should have meat in their diet. My argument would then be, perhaps we should not breed and keep domestic dogs and cats. For when cats go feral, due to human neglect, they become the biggest killers of our natural wildlife[11]. And dogs gone wild collect into packs and become a menace to wildlife and people in rural areas too. Australia alone has such a huge wild dog problem that the government has no idea how to deal with it (If this is topic that interests you I highly recommend Guy Hull's *The Dogs that Made*

---

[11] https://invasives.org.au/blog/meet-the-27-native-animals-cats-have-helped-send-extinct-since-colonisation/

Australia)[12]. In Australia alone, it is estimated that cats are responsible for sixty-five per cent of all indigenous species extinction, and both free ranging domestic and feral cats kill up to two billion native animals every year. And of course, we are directly implicated in that loss of beauty and diversity, because we breed and sell these killers.

Ownership of any animal is really a contentious issue. I live in a small town neighbourhood in rural New South Wales, Australia, where the local dogs bark incessantly at the slightest noise, at each other, and it would seem, at almost anything. Why, because they are bored senseless, like a bear in a zoo cage and an enclosure that is way too small for its big body. They want to get out and run, and chase cats, and get into a pack and pull down big animals. Unless of course we spend our time with them, walk them and nurture them, and then they become a part of the family. But we have to work at this; we can't just have a pet and then expect it to be happy just because we feed it. Ownership of an animal, should we decide this is what we want to do with our spare time, requires effort, love and commitment. But, in the long term, it is a difficult subject to navigate, because of the nature of where all our pets come from. My opinion is that we either have fully vegan-fed pets, or we learn to live without them, because we cannot have a vegan world with slaughter as part of that world. The cycle of destruction has to come to an end somehow and at some point in time. Maybe you have a better answer than I have come up with? That is part of my hope for this book, that the vegan solutionaries that are rising in this world today are the very people that will solve the many animal abuse problems

[12] www.amazon.com.au/Dogs-that-Made-Australia-Transformation/dp/1460756452

we live with today. I have faith that you are out there now, waiting for your day. Wait no longer, your day has come, and I hope that I live long enough to meet some of you and thank you personally for your great work.

Ethical Leadership: The Solutionaries are Rising

"I am in favor of animal rights as well as human rights. That is the way of a whole human being." Abraham Lincoln (1809–1865)

It is almost impossible to write about veganism without addressing the subject of ethical leadership. This is something that I have been alluding to since the beginning of the book; these are the very 'solutionaries' that I have been talking about. Those courageous people from all walks of life who are beginning to see, not only the direction we need to go in as a species for our planet, but are coming forward with solutions to carry these ideas to fruition. Let us hope that with wisdom and ethics on our side, the world will pull together to make the necessary changes possible.

I do not want to focus on any one political party, but moreover simply to look at what it looks like to be an ethical leader. There are in the world today, a growing number of ordinary people bringing new and extraordinary ideas to the table of politics and leadership. They are doing this with wisdom, clarity and ethics that defies and challenges the status quo of the old adage of 'more the same'. Many of these new leaders are young women with the vigour of youth on their side and a deep and ethical vibrancy to challenge the tired old white men, who seem to have what looks like a stranglehold on keeping things just as they are. I would say that it is not enough to simply be vegan, although that is a great place to start, but to be truly ethical in the face of the political colossus we all face, one must be prepared to live and breathe the ethics that change requires.

We simply cannot go on living in the world as we do today, and expect to survive. The change required is immeasurably larger and more demanding than it has ever been in recorded history. For an ethical leader to not only survive these larger than life challenges, they must also be prepared to not water down their ethics by doing deals with other, let us say, less than ethical political parties. It is important to remember the political statement from Jerry Garcia that suggests, when we are 'constantly choosing the lesser of two evils [it] is still choosing evil'. If we really want to see real and lasting change in this world of suffering, then we have to follow in the footsteps of all of history's greatest examples and lead with compassion, kindness and what in Sanskrit is called 'Ahimsa', which is defined as the principle of non-injury to living beings. We simply cannot continue to trade in living beings, without the consequential abuse and injury we cause by doing so. The world needs to prepare itself for really big changes.

Thus, when deals are done between political parties, the principle of, 'you scratch my back, and I'll scratch yours'', simply won't work if it is the ethical change we wish to see. This sort of dealmaking not only waters down the ethics we live for and wish to see unfolding within our world. It also inadvertently undoes the good we have so far achieved and makes our strong and powerful arguments of real, true and lasting ethical change seem weak and insipid. We are, as it were, selling our soul to the devil every time we do this. This is going to take courage of a new ethical symetry to break through into the fresh ground of a peaceful world. Where the unnecessary and abysmally unethical behaviour of most political parties and their corporate funders will begin to fall short and their attempts to continue to dominate will be overturned by the ethics of kindess over profit.

I believe that the dawning of a new age of ethical and compassionate leadership is about to be born – this is needed more than anything else right now: we need a world where leaders make choices based on a love for all life, not just on human centred economic structures. If leadership comes from a deep place of compassion we can only steer a steady course towards a beautiful life for all sentient beings. I truly believe that our duty of care to all living beings in this world is *not* to enjoy them on our taste buds but to love them all, each and everyone, as if they were our very own children. What a beautiful world that would be to live in. One of the best books on this subject to date is *Golden Age Politics*[13] by Kathy Divine. The book explores the many aspects of ethical leadership and I am sure it will inspire many to take up the challenge of our age.

I will leave you with my personal musing on this subject; as this is what I believe may help bring clarity in its simplest form. The world we are told is complex, but the world is not complex, we have made it complex, and we need to get back to some fundamental principles of ethical behaviour. And to do this, we need to keep it simple:

My idea is that the universe itself is *Love*; this is how Einstein, Gandhi and others have described it. Thus, if we live in accordance with this knowledge, we begin to practise *Peace* in our everyday lives, and our thoughts, actions and intentions are filled with the peaceful love of the Universe. The result of living this way leads directly to *Harmony* on every level of our lives, and there can be no other result while we

---

[13] www.amazon.com.au/Golden-Age-Politics-Inspired-Peaceful/dp/0994446225

continue to recognise that *Love* is the most powerful force in the Universe.

If we can live by the simplicity of these ideas, the rising solutionary leaders of our world, many of whom probably already live this way, will continue to lead the way towards a brighter, healthier, more compassionate, and certainly kinder future for all life on our planet.

Innate Psychological Health and Wellbeing

"The secret to happiness is not to go out there and try and find it. Because happiness is not out there. Happiness is within the consciousness of every human being." Sydney Banks (1931–2009)

This leads on to a subject close to my heart, which is our innate mental health and psychological wellbeing. For a short while in the 1980's, I was chair of a small animal rights group based in the UK. Despite my most fervent efforts, I could not continue with this work due to the simple fact that almost every member of the group that attended meetings were in some way shape or form, depressed by the overwhelming consequences of knowing what they knew about the treatment and suffering of animals the world over. This may seem understandable at first view, but it certainly gave me food for thought.

I didn't have the answers I needed at the time to help these beautiful people, and so I had to give it up as a bad job. I really wanted to help them move on and feel better in themselves, but I just didn't have the skill set to really help them get out of the thinking that so often goes with the territory of dwelling on animal suffering. Now, I would do things very differently and feel confident that I could help almost any individual or group find a deeper sense of peace of mind to live from.

Now I am confident that I could give any working group a gentle guiding hand back towards the power that each individual has inside of them. That may sound like a pretentious statement, but I am happy to be put to the test. I love a good challenge. I am happy to work with any animal rights group, ethical political party, or any organisation that is endeavouring to do this great work to alleviate and prevent the suffering of the beautiful animals of our world.

New Thoughts

"There is a road from the eye to the heart that does not go through the intellect." G. K. Chesterton (1874–1936)

A good number of years back I was giving a talk at the London Vegan Fair. When the time came for questions and answers I was asked one incredibly interesting question about thought. What I had suggested to the audience was that it was the way we were seeing the world that made us feel the way we felt, not the circumstances that we were witnessing as evident in the world today. The woman's question went something like this: "I understand what you mean about our positive mental attitude[14], and personal thinking, as I am okay most of the time, but don't you know that there are millions of animals suffering all over the world, I'm not sure if you realise that, so how can thought help with that?"

My suggestion to her and the audience at large was that despite the known fact (that I was very well aware of), that there are indeed

[14] Please note I was in no way suggesting the practice of 'positive thinking', which as anyone who has attempted it, will know, only lasts as long as you have positive thoughts. As a technique, like most techniques, it is dead in the water.

millions of animals suffering and dying around the world on a daily basis, that this fact had nothing to do with our mental attitude. Additionally, I suggested that as a known fact, which was easily verifiable to be true, it still didn't mean we had to automatically remain angry, or upset or depressed by this knowledge all the time. Initially, of course our compassionate response might be to be saddened and upset by such knowledge, and by all means angered. Yet, the only way we could continue to feel these unsettling feelings would be to continue to think about the suffering and consequently the solution would elude us. If we find ourselves focusing only on the thing that upsets us then as a consequence, we are not really looking for the solution. This is due to the simple fact that we cannot do both things at the same time. Creativity and solutions to problems don't usually tend to arise in an unhappy or low thinking blinkered mind.

I suggested that if our mind was clear and neutral then, we would more likely be in a much stronger position to access the common sense and wisdom required to come up with the very solution we were looking for. And that this solution would continue to evade us while we remained in an angry or low feeling state, created via our thinking. This is due to the fact that while we are in a negative state of mind our thinking becomes narrow and blinkered and it becomes impossible to continue to see the bigger picture. This can happen to all of us, no one is totally immune; yet seeing the bigger picture is where all the solutions to the world's problems lie. In the quiet stillness of our own minds lies all the answers to all of the problems we face in the world today, if we can get quiet enough to see them. In fact I would add that there are no problems as such, simply solutions waiting to be discovered when we get quiet enough to hear them.

Common Sense, Creativity and Wisdom

"You put a baby in a crib with an apple and a rabbit. If it eats the rabbit and plays with the apple, I'll buy you a new car." Harvey Diamond (1945–)

Listening to our common sense and wisdom, and using our creativity is where our true power lies. We always, always have the power of common sense, creativity and innate wisdom within us. We were born with it, and this innate health can never be taken away from us, or damaged in any way. We can of course cover it over with our personal and conditioned thinking, but that means that it is always sitting just below the surface of our current and in-the-moment thinking. Sometimes people ask me, how do we know when we are experiencing wisdom or common sense? My reply has always been the same for many years now; we know when it is wisdom because it always comes with a deep sense of certainty, a profound knowing that comes from within us, and not from our memories or conditioned thoughts. We could say that this feeling of self-assurance is also a good feeling.

Can you see where I am going with this? And how this could help anyone with ears to listen with an open mind. We do not have to be trapped or held down by our thinking about what we know to be happening to animals out there in the world. In fact we can set ourselves free from ongoing pain that so many suffer from simply by understanding what the Buddha once suggested: 'It is our mind that creates this world'. If we can really see this, that the 'reality' that we are currently experiencing (in this very moment as you read these words), is all coming from within, then we are free to experience a new reality. A new reality where we become the very solution we have been looking for for so long. I think for many people they perhaps always thought that solutions lay outside of themselves, somewhere out there in the world. Freedom, true psychological freedom comes from within, not from something on the outside of us. As I stated much earlier in this book, you could be the very person that comes up with the solution we have all been waiting for, and from there, all the magic will unfold and a new history of ethics will be born. I am certain we all want that ethicl and kinder world to come sooner rather than later.

Making a Difference in the World

"Whenever you find yourself on the side of the majority, it's time to pause and reflect." Mark Twain (1835–1910)

If we really want to make a difference in this world for our beautiful cousins of the animal kingdom, and there are, of course, many paths we can take to do this, but the best and most useful preparation is to have a quiet mind. There is a simple logic to the mind, and it is this, whatever kind of thought we are having is all that we can experience in the living moment. A thought enters our mind and consciousness makes it appear real to us. In other words, we have a loving thought, we feel loving feelings, we have an angry thought, and we feel angry feelings. There really is no other way our mind can work. Thus the reality we feel and experience around us is created via our own thinking. Life isn't happening to us, we are living in the world, and life appears as it does, dependent on the current state of our thinking. What I am talking about is that, put simply, our experience comes from the way we are seeing our universe. We create our moment-to-moment reality from the inside, not the other way around. Another way of explaining this would be to see how our moods change. Moods go up and they go down. Why do they do this? Again, it is simply the direction our thinking has taken us. I defy anyone who can remain in a low mood forever. For once something or someone has distracted us away from the thinking that had created the low feelings in the first place, we simply return to our natural state, which is a state of *beautiful neutrality*. Of course we can simply go back to the previous thinking and engage in low feeling once more, however, when we see that this is where all of our feelings are coming from, it becomes much harder to maintain a low state of mind. This is due to the simple fact that we begin to recognise that it is our thinking that is creating these feelings of going up and down and not as we might have previously believed, that it was somehow coming from the world and from our current circumstances.

A Quiet Mind

"Learn to be silent. Let your quiet mind listen and absorb."
Pythagoras (570–490 BCE)

When our mind becomes quiet, even for a millisecond, wisdom fills the gap. It's just that living as we do, in this age of absolute information overload, we become saturated with ideas, concepts, theories, and opinions. If we add all of this information to the conditioned thinking we already have inside us, as part of who we think we are, we start to see the potential for utter confusion. We grow up and become a product of our conditioning, that is to say, all we have ever read in books, magazines, newspapers, and everything we have ever heard and seen through television, movies, or podcasts, not the least our parenting, education system and conversations with each other. This is how we end up seeing the world through that lens which is somewhat misted and cloudy. Rather, the quiet still voice of wisdom brings us the clarity to see the world around us without the lens of our conditioning getting in the way.

How is this possible you may ask? And how do we access our natural innate intelligence and wisdom? As mentioned before, it comes from having a quiet mind. Think of it like this; when we listen to music, we don't generally try to analyse the sounds, we simply enjoy them. Likewise when viewing visual art, we look and take in the beauty, the colours and the images, without the need to evaluate or scrutinise. These are aesthetic experiences. Again with theatre, or movies, we 'suspend disbelief' for the duration of the experience, usually without the desire to appraise. In nature, our greatest teacher, when we find ourselves in awe of a beautiful scene of a mountain, dell or beachscape, or a sunset or rainbow, mostly the last thing on our mind is some form of analytical judgement. We simply luxuriate and swim in these fleeting magical experiences. These are all examples when the mind sees the world around us, without the filter and lens of conditioning. We could call it the gap between thoughts, and this is where wisdom shows itself.

No doubt many of you have heard the derogatory statement: "Oh, that person just sees the world through rose tinted lenses!" I often wonder what colour the lenses are of the people asking this innocently prejudiced question? I think the impression is that these people with rosy tinted lenses are somehow seeing a distorted view of reality, and the questioner is somehow seeing the 'real world'. However, what is really happening is that we all live in our bubble, our own version of reality made up of our conditioning as mentioned above. Think about this for a moment, if every single person on the planet is creating their own personal version of reality, is it any wonder, we end up confused in communication with each other at times. It is what is known as living in a separate reality, and we all have our very own personal version.

The 'Aha' Moments

"The intuitive mind is a sacred gift and the rational mind is a faithful servant. We have created a society that honors the servant and has forgotten the gift." Albert Einstein (1879–1955)

How many times have you been trying to think of a word, or a name of someone during a conversation, and you cannot find it for love nor money while 'trying' to do so. Yet, once you have moved on, stopped trying and simply got on with your day, the very thing or word, or name you so desperately searched for is right in your mind. This is wisdom, common sense, and intuition. Thus, if we are trying hard to relax the mind, to be at peace to find the very wisdom that lies deep within us all, which is always just one thought away, we need to let go of the trying and let wisdom arise without effort. Another example is when there is a puzzle or problem in our mind, and we just can't find the answers for the solution. Then, more often than not, we get our answers when we are not looking for them, and it can literally be anywhere, the shower, driving to the store, daydreaming while looking out a window, or even doing housework. It is in these moments when the intellect is switched to 'off' mode, free flowing and not perusing the memory banks of our conditioning, that wisdom has a chance to breakthrough to the surface, and 'boom', there is our answer. I would add here that literally all of the problems and questions that life might throw our way have a corresponding answer, if we are quiet enough inside to hear them.

I would like to make a distinction here between reason, and wisdom, because what some call 'reason' is really just a collection of ideas or concepts that are again based on an intellectual understanding of the world via our conditioning. That is not what I mean by wisdom. What I am talking about here in terms of wisdom is our innate ability to know wrong from right, our intuition, our common sense, our gut instinct to use a few frequently used terms. Wisdom, as Sydney Banks[15] often suggested, always, always comes with a good feeling. And as mentioned before, I would add that it also comes with a deep sense of certainty, confidence and a knowing. It appears at those times when we simply *know* what direction we must go in and how to proceed in life with a definite certitude.

Genius

"Genius is nothing more nor less than childhood recaptured at will."
Charles Baudelaire (1821–1867)

As I used to say to many of my high school students: "Did you know you were all born with genius inside of you, and you all have enough wisdom to get you through your entire life, whatever anyone says about you?" More often than not the students would reply: "Oh no sir, you've got the wrong class, we're all thick in here." My reply was always the same, I would tell them that I was not talking about so-called 'book learning', but the wisdom and innate intelligence that we are all born with. I really wanted them to know, as I do you my reader, that there is no one alive with an ounce more wisdom than you were born with. It is just that more often than not people struggle to access it, or think that it comes with age, or practice or that it is in some way, outside of them in the world. When in fact it has been on the very end of our nose since the day we were born. All the sages and spiritual leaders since the beginning of time have all endeavoured to point people to their own innate wisdom. Rarely

---

[15] https://sydbanks.com/

claiming to be the expert, but moreover, the mirror to show us our own inner worth and wisdom.

Conclusion

I hope by now you will see that what I am pointing towards is that our deep and abiding capacity for good and wonderful deeds, can only be made stronger by truly understanding our amazing ability to return to wisdom via a quiet mind. I fully appreciate that an intellectual understanding of what I am saying here is of very little use to anyone. It is what my gran used to call a 'chocolate teapot'; add boiling water to it and all we have is a big mess to clean up. The intellect is our brain power, and can be added to, enhanced by study and aided by discussion, but our innate wisdom is our inborn capacity and a power of an even greater magnitude, because it is of the spirit, and is ultimately what really drives us to great deeds of love and compassion.

My hope is that somewhere in your consciousness you will find the natural ability to read, not just between the lines, the magic of who you really are, beyond the words themselves to the Oneness of Life. Which is what, and who we really are at an energetic level. We are, I once heard it suggested: *"the Universe itself, given eyes, and looking back at itself in awe and wonder"*. If we can let go of all that we think we are, even for a fraction of a second, then, what we will see will change us forever. For time itself is the great illusion, and the wisdom we speak of here is outside of time altogether.

This journey is a voyage of love and forgiveness: love, because it is the most powerful force in the known universe, and as such we will do so much more good with love in our hearts than anything else. And forgiveness, because along the way, if we are to have the most impact upon this world of suffering, we are going to have to learn to forgive the people that are blind to all the animal suffering in the world. If we cannot forgive, we will harbour hidden resentment and even anger, and this will never help to end the perpetual cycle of suffering.

I wish you all a wonderful journey towards a deeper life of compassion, ethics and love. Have the best life ever, for as we are told, life is but short and sweet and must be lived to the fullest.

I will leave you with the words of one of my favourite poets:

"What is it you plan to do with your one wild and precious life?" Mary Oliver (1935–2019)

Further Reading

Sydney Banks, *Second Chance,* Duval-Bibb Publsihing, 1989

Sydney Banks, *In search of the Pearl*, Duval-Bibb Publsihing, 1990

Sydney Banks, *The Missing Link*, International Human Relations Consultants Inc, 1998

Sydney Banks, *The Enlightened Gardener*, International Human Relations Consultants Inc, 2001

Sydney Banks, *Dear Liza*, Lone Pine Publishing, 2004

Sydney Banks, *The Enlightened Gardener Revisited*, Lone Pine Publishing, 2005

T. Colin Campbell, Thomas M. Campbell, *The China Study*, Benbella Books, 2004

Kathy Divine, *Vegans Are Cool*, Createspace Publishing, 2013

Kathy Divine, *Plant Powered Men,* Createspace Publishing, 2013

Kathy Divine, *Plant Powered Women*, Createspace Publishing, 2013

Kathy Divine, *Golden Age Politics*, Peace Era Publishing, 2020

Gary L. Francione, Anna Charlton, *Eat Like You Care: An Examination of the Morality of Eating Animals*, Createspace, 2013

Michael Greger MD, Gene Stone, *How Not to Die: Discover the Foods Scientifically Proven to Prevent and Reverse Disease*, Flairton Books, 2015

Melanie Joy, *Why We Love Dogs, Eat Pigs and Wear Cows: An Introduction to Carnism,* Conairy Press US, 2011

Tobias Leenaert, *How to Create a Vegan World: A Pragmatic Approach*, Lantern Books US, 2017

Clare Mann, *Vystopia: The Anguish at Being Vegan in a Non-Vegans World*, Communicate31 Pty Ltd, 2018

Jack Pransky, *Modello: A Story of Hope for the Inner City and Beyond,* CCB Publishing, 2011

Dean Rees-Evans, *The Great Remebering: Turning the world Insideout,* Three Principles Press, 2021

Peter Singer, *Why Vegan*, Liveright Publishers, 2020

Peter Singer, *Animal Liberation*, HarperCollins Publishers Inc, 2009

Colin Tuge, *The Secret Life of Trees*, Penguin Press, 2006

Peter Tomkins, Christopher Bird, *The Secret Life of Plants*, Howe & Row, 1973

Flavia Ursino-Coleman, *Beyond Speicisim*, USNCOL Pty. Ltd, 2020

Zoe Weil, *Most Good, Least Harm*, Simon & Schuster, 2009

Peter Wholleben, *The Hidden Life of Trees: What they Feel, How they Communicate*, Greystone Books, 2016

My dictionary definitions

annibalism

[**an**-*uh-buh-liz-uh* m]

noun

1. the eating of flesh by a human being.
2. the eating of flesh of an animal by another animal of its own world or planet with enough intelligence to comprehend the unnecessity of it.
3. the ceremonial eating of flesh or parts of an animal's body for magical, religious or cultural purposes, as to acquire the power or skill of an animal recently killed.
4. the act of eating flesh with the misguided belief that it is required for protein or health

vevolution

[veev-*uh*-**loo**-sh*uh*n]

noun

1. any process of formation or growth; development: *the evolution of the human mind; the evolution of the way we eat.*

2. a product of such development; something evolved: *The exploration of diet and nutrition is the evolution of decades of research.*

3. *Biology.* Change in the gene pool of a population from generation to generation by such processes as mutation, natural selection, and genetic drift: *Humans begin to realise that eating meat is antiquated.*

4. a process of gradual, peaceful, progressive change or development, as in social or economic structure or institutions. *Humans begin to see that compassion and ethics are more important than profit.*

5. a motion incomplete in itself, but combining with coordinated motions to produce a single action, as in a machine: *Such as the desire in humans to shut down the mechanisms of the globalised killing machines to end animal suffering for good.*

Dean's Organic Vegan Curry Recipe

Ingredients:

- 3 or 4 large onions or bunches of spring onions (medium chopped).
- 3 or 4 cloves of garlic or garlic powder (finely chopped or crushed).
- 2 large cauliflowers (finely chopped into very small florets).
- 1 bag of potatoes (cut into small cubes).
- 1 large bunch of carrots (topped and tailed, cut diagonally along the carrot & then cut into chip like pieces – *this is essential for flavour*).
- a mixture of any other seasonal veg you would like (French green beans, peas, sweet corn, broccoli, cabbage, etc.)
- 1 or 2 large cartons of mushrooms (sliced or quartered or half and half)
- 1 & half cups of dried chickpeas/garbanzo beans cooked in advance (or a tin of the equivalent).
- 1 & half cups of dried mixed beans or butter beans, red kidney, black eye/ black beans cooked in advance (or the equivalent in tinned).
- 500 grams of red lentils (or tinned).
- 3 or 4 Vegetable stock cubes (finely chopped).
- 1 large tablespoonful of Marmite/vegemite/yeast extract (dissolved in a little water or in the curry mixture) use more if you need to.
- 1 large tablespoonful or more of Peanut or any nut butter (dissolved in a little water or in the curry mixture).

- 1 block of creamed coconut or from a jar (cut into small pieces).
- 1 tin of coconut cream (full fat)

Spices:

- Curry (medium/hot or Madras) powder
- Coriander powder
- Coriander leaf (dried)
- Ground cumin seeds
- Chilli powder
- Turmeric powder
- Ginger powder
- Paprika powder
- Poppy seeds
- Garam masala
- 2 or 3 teaspoons of Sea salt
- Tamari to taste

Preparation:

- Steam the cauliflower, put into a bowl once cooked, ready for the mixture.
- Steam the potatoes, carrots and any other veg ready for the mixture, place in a bowl.
- Fry the onions first then add the mushrooms into the bottom of a large pan suitable for cooking the curry in.
- When the mushrooms are slightly browned add some cold water and mix in well, being sure to get all the cooked flavour from the bottom of the pan into the mix of water (you can do this with the frying pan too).

- Add all the vegetables to the pan with some of the stock water from the steamer.
- Cover the surface of the veg mix with curry powder (don't be shy now, use plenty)
- Add the stock cubes
- Add the marmite/vegemite
- Add the Tamari
- Add the peanut butter
- Add the creamed coconut & the coconut cream/milk
- Add the sea salt
- Add a good amount of poppy seeds
- Add all the spices to taste (don't be shy with them)
- Note: (If you don't have a steamer, cook the veg in a big pot with less water and fry the onions and mushrooms in a frying pan and add later)

Then stir, stir, stir – if it looks dry add some Coconut, almond, oat or soy milk to keep it moving.

Serve with wholegrain Basmati Rice, Quinoa, or another grain and enjoy!

Keep in mind that you have a lot of veg in there; if you taste it and it seems too mild or too bland, add more Tamari, Marmite and curry powder, or any of the herbs and spices you like, then try it again until it tastes as you like it.

My dear friend Marion once cooked it for me when I was recovering from surgery, when we sat down to eat I exclaimed: "Wow, it tastes just like when I cook it!" She looked surprised, and replied: "Well, I did follow the recipe".

Happy cooking and enjoy the feast

Acknowledgments

Firstly I would like to thank all of the vegan authors out there in the world that laid down a clear and ethical path to live from, this book would not perhaps, have been possible without them.

And my heartfelt thanks goes to all my review readers, you have all been kind in your appraisal of my book: Lea McBride, Kathy Divine, Avleen Masawan, Kimberley Deeney, Dhammakumara, Robyn Chuter, Jennie Fenton, Tracey Chapman, Anne Bates, Flavia Ursino Coleman, Clare Mann, and Bob Ratnaraja.

Additionally, a special mention and thanks for Doug and Alyson Blackwell; for their early reading of the text and invaliuable feedback on the manuscript. Also a big thank you to my editors, firstly Naomi Elliot for her clear thinking guidence and comments on the text, and to Tom Rothsey for an invaluable last minute critical review and editorial suggestions, the book is much the better for it.

And finally, I endeavour to remind myself that every book is a collaboration, for without the help of a community of friends and colleauges the dream of a book may remain just that. Thank you all from the bottom of my heart.

Dean Rees-Evans MSc - March 2023

About the Author

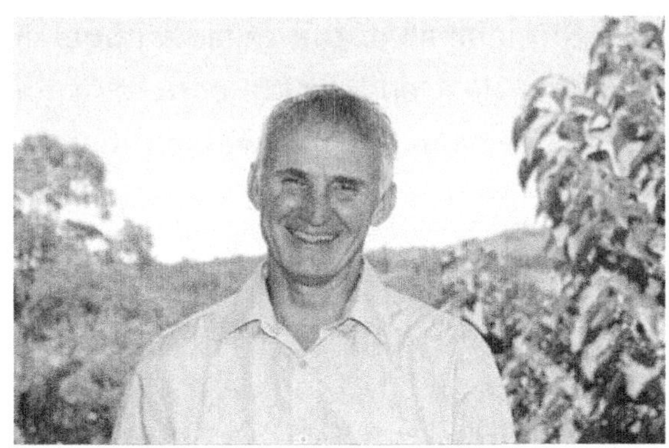

Dean Rees-Evans MSc is a Human Relations Consultant, mentor, teacher, researcher, international public speaker and author. After completing training in 2004 with the eminent Californian psychologist, the late Dr. Roger Mills, and Mr Sydney Banks Dean has been mentoring individuals, couples, families and conducts trainings in schools, hospitals and business. He has extensive experience with teenagers and is author his first book: *The Great Remembering: Turning the World Inside out*, a well-being book for teens of all ages.

Dean received his MSc after conducting a successful research pilot study at a UK high school working with both staff and pupils. The *Three Principles* is a dynamic, insight-based approach that focuses upon the natural and innate health that lies within all humans. Dean's pioneering research revealed increases in psychological happiness and well-being of a highly significant nature.

Establishing ***Three Principles: Well-Being for Life*** in 2005, he conducts inspiring and life-changing workshops, offers dynamic individual and group mentoring and holds uplifting public events. Connect with Dean via social media and his website to keep informed about his work.

facebook.com/ThreePrinciplesTraining

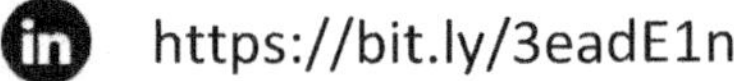

threeprinciples.com.au

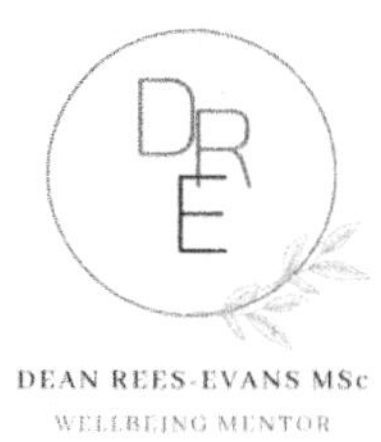

Printed in Great Britain
by Amazon